WHO Manual for the standardized investigation, diagnosis and management of the infertile male

The treatment of male infertility has been revolutionized by advances in assisted reproductive technology. This concise and structured account, prepared by an authoritative international panel of experts, provides a consensus on the most effective and logical approach to the investigation and management of male infertility. It focuses attention on three key areas: history-taking; clinical assessment of male fertility; and objective criteria for diagnostic categories. This approach complements the areas covered in the companion volume *WHO Laboratory Manual for the Examination of Human Semen and Sperm–Cervical Mucus Interaction* (CUP, 4th edn, 1999) and significantly expands upon the section on male infertility in the previous volume on the infertile couple *WHO Manual for the Standardized Investigation and Diagnosis of the Infertile Couple* (CUP, 1993). This new, practical consensus will be an indispensable guide to good clinical management of all forms of male infertility.

T0236599

WHO MANUAL

for the standardized investigation, diagnosis and management of the infertile male

Patrick J. Rowe

World Health Organization
Geneva, Switzerland

Frank H. Comhaire

University Hospital
Ghent, Belgium

Timothy B. Hargreave

University of Edinburgh
Edinburgh, Scotland

Ahmed M. A. Mahmoud

University Hospital
Ghent, Belgium

Published on behalf of the
WORLD HEALTH ORGANIZATION
by

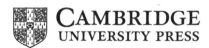
CAMBRIDGE
UNIVERSITY PRESS

CAMBRIDGE
UNIVERSITY PRESS

University Printing House, Cambridge CB2 8BS, United Kingdom

Cambridge University Press is part of the University of Cambridge.

It furthers the University's mission by disseminating knowledge in the pursuit of education, learning and research at the highest international levels of excellence.

www.cambridge.org
Information on this title: www.cambridge.org/9780521774741

First published 2000
Reprinted 2003

A catalogue record for this publication is available from the British Library

ISBN 978-0-521-77474-1 Paperback

Cambridge University Press has no responsibility for the persistence or accuracy of URLs for external or third-party internet websites referred to in this publication, and does not guarantee that any content on such websites is, or will remain, accurate or appropriate.

....

Contents

Preface

While it is imperative that each case of infertility is considered clinically as a couple, evolution in our management of the male and female partners proceeds asynchronously. Since publication of the first edition of the *WHO Manual for the Standardized Investigation, Diagnosis and Management of the Infertile Couple* in 1993 there have been major developments in our ability to help couples with a significant male factor achieve a pregnancy. Many of these treatment options involve the use of assisted reproductive technology, ranging from intrauterine insemination to in vitro fertilization and even intracytoplasmic sperm injection for the most severe cases. Less dramatic progress has been made in developing more successful treatment options for couples with female factors.

Consequently, while there is a clear need to revise and update that part of the Manual concerning the male partner, the section on the female partner requires little change. Therefore it was decided to divide the Manual into two volumes. This was not an easy decision and must not be taken as any indication of a move away from considering infertility as a problem of a couple, it is purely a pragmatic publishing decision.

The present Manual has been approved by consensus reached among the authors and an international board of experts.

International board of experts

1 Introduction

The term infertility is used to describe the situation where a couple does not succeed in achieving a spontaneous pregnancy in spite of the 'exposure to the risk of pregnancy' during a given period of time (see The definition of infertility, p. 5). Infertility may be either permanent and irreversible, e.g. in many cases of azoospermia, and is then referred to as 'sterility', or the probability of spontaneous conception may be decreased, but not reduced to zero, when the term 'subfertility' is used.

Traditionally, the female partner is held responsible for the failure to conceive. However, in reality, male reproductive capacity was found to be deficient in not less than 50% of infertile couples evaluated according to a study by the World Health Organization (1987). Evaluation of the male should take place with each couple coming to the consultation for infertility, and it must be performed at the beginning of their investigation. Indeed, male investigation is easy, cheap and painless and it will result rapidly in diagnostic categorization (as listed in Table 1.1). It is recommended that a complete diagnostic profile be reached for each individual patient by marking the logic path on the flowchart. Several causal diagnoses may be present simultaneously. The diagnostic classification aims at therapeutic strategies rather than at academically detailed subclassification that has no direct impact on clinical management.

The *WHO Manual* also provides general guidelines to the management of the infertile couple with a male factor. It should be kept in mind that male subfertility is commonly associated with one or more factors that decrease the probability of conception in the female partner (see Diagnostic categories and management, p. 37). Correction of such factors in the female partner must always be performed in parallel with treatment of the male

Table 1.1. *Male diagnostic categories*

Sexual and/or ejaculatory dysfunction
Immunological cause
No demonstrable abnormality
Isolated seminal plasma abnormalities
Iatrogenic cause
Systemic cause
Congenital abnormalities

1. Testicular maldescent
2. Karyotype abnormalities
3. Congenital agenesis of the seminal vesicles and/or vasa deferentia
   (a cause of obstructive azoospermia)
4. Other congenital diseases

Acquired testicular damage
Varicocele
Male accessory gland infection
Endocrine cause
Idiopathic oligozoospermia
Idiopathic asthenozoospermia
Idiopathic teratozoospermia
Idiopathic cryptozoospermia
Obstructive azoospermia
Idiopathic azoospermia

partner, and the couple must be counselled on the diagnostic procedures and therapeutic options. Counselling must also aim at relieving tensions and anxiety which commonly occur during the investigation and management of infertility (Felder et al., 1996).

The choice of treatment must be based on considerations of evidence-based medicine as well as on cost-effectiveness estimates, but must also take into account the ethical, religious and emotional views of the couple themselves. From the ethical point of view, the non-maleficence principle (*primum non nocere* or first do no harm) must be rigorously adhered to, and great care must be taken not to induce any pathology in the mother or the offspring.

It should be remembered that the success of treating male infertility can only be evaluated indirectly through the occurrence of pregnancy in the female partner. Since the latter commonly presents with decreased fertility, it is extremely difficult to prove the effectiveness of particular treatments of the male partner. Nevertheless, meta-analyses of controlled studies, prospective cohort studies, and – more significantly – several prospective randomized trials have been undertaken, yielding results that have clinical relevance.

The implementation of evidence-based medicine in reproductive medicine, particularly in the diagnosis and management of the infertile male, poses major problems (Comhaire, 1998).

- Few recommendations can be categorized as 'definite' being based on evidence from highly reliable clinical research.
- The majority of recommendations are based on the results of meta-analyses and of reliable cohort studies. In the text these are described as: 'generally accepted'.
- When a particular approach is controversial, the following terminologies are used: 'some authors suggest/believe' or 'it has been reported'. In these situations, references are given to support the viewpoint.

In formulating these guidelines for the management of the infertile couple, the authors have relied mainly on the results of controlled prospective studies performed under supervision of WHO. The authors are aware of the fact that other studies may have come to different conclusions. Also, the general guidelines for management must be applied in a judicious manner adapted to the specific situation of any individual couple, taking into account complementary factors such as duration of infertility, and age of both partners especially that of the female.

2 History-taking

The principal reason for history-taking is that it will contribute to the diagnosis in one-quarter of cases of infertility. It also helps to define the prognosis and will influence decisions about management (Abramsson et al., 1989; Micic, 1987; Collins et al., 1984).

It takes time to take a full history and it is easy to forget items. The WHO scheme (Appendix I) is a structured interview, which allows relevant information to be obtained and makes best use of time. Some clinics may find it useful to send the patient a questionnaire prior to the first visit, but this may not be appropriate in all countries.

Although it is helpful to interview the couple together for history-taking, there may be some questions that are better asked when the man is alone, for example, history of previous sexual partners, pregnancies, sexually transmitted disease, etc. These questions can be asked conveniently at the same time as physical examination is performed.

The following text explains the WHO definitions used during the standard investigation of the male partner. Where appropriate, comments are made about the clinical or scientific significance of each item.

2.1 THE DEFINITION OF INFERTILITY

Infertility is defined as no conception after at least 12 months of unprotected intercourse. The time limit of 12 months is arbitrary, but corresponds with the fact that the majority (approximately 85%) of couples who achieve pregnancy spontaneously will do so within 12 months. This does not imply, however, that investigation for infertility must be postponed until the period of 12 months has elapsed, particularly if the couple has familial

Table 2.1. *Cumulated conception probability for the most recent TTP of the couple (age adjusted)*

Region	Cumulated conception probability (%) at			Planned pregnancy (%)	Number of couples
	6 months	12 months	24 months		
Denmark	66	74	79	79	714
Germany, West	62	74	80	67	697
Germany, East	63	74	83	69	460
Poland	45	54	64	51	365
Italy, North	61	73	79	72	1241
Italy, South	79	87	89	90	623
Spain	77	84	88	83	685
Total	65	75	81	74	4785

Note:
TTP = time to pregnancy.
Source: Adapted from Juul et al., 1997, permission requested.

reasons or events in their history to suspect infertility in either partner. A recent study involving five European countries indicated regional variations in cumulative pregnancy rates (Table 2.1) (Juul, 1997).

2.1.1 Primary male infertility

This is when the man has never impregnated a women.

2.1.2 Impregnation

Impregnation is when a man initiated a pregnancy, independent of the outcome of that pregnancy.

2.1.3 Secondary male infertility

This is when the man has impregnated a women, irrespective of whether she is the present partner and irrespective of the outcome of the pregnancy. Men with secondary infertility, in general, have a better chance of future fertility. Also, certain diagnoses are less likely to be found, such as congenital disorders or severe impairment of sperm production with azoospermia or extreme oligozoospermia, whereas varicocele and, perhaps, male accessory gland infection are more common (Robertson & Harrison, 1984). In men with secondary infertility, histories of certain treatments or exposure to toxic agents, such as X-rays,

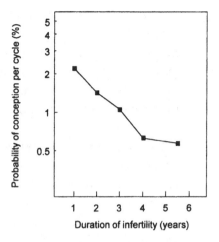

Fig. 2.1. The probability of conception per cycle of exposure (P/C) is shown in relation to the duration of infertility. Note that P/C values are plotted on a logarithmic scale (adapted from Comhaire, 1996; WHO, 1984).

benzenes, or pesticides, are risk factors for azoospermia (Thonneau et al., 1983).

2.1.4 The duration of involuntary infertility

This is defined as the number of months during which the couple has been having sexual intercourse without the use of any contraceptive method. This is important as it gives prognostic information about the couple's future fertility. Those couples with a duration of infertility of approximately 3 years or less have a better chance of future spontaneous pregnancy (Fig. 2.1). If the duration of involuntary infertility has been longer, then it is likely that there is a severe biological problem.

The duration of infertility is important when designing or reporting clinical and scientific studies of infertility. In uncontrolled clinical trials the spontaneous pregnancy rate may be misinterpreted as a treatment effect.

In general, couples in developed countries tend to seek medical advice after a shorter duration of infertility. The duration of involuntary infertility gives no information about whether the problem is with the male or the female partner.

In cases of secondary infertility the months since the last impregnation should be noted (see p. 6 for definition). For men with secondary infertility, this is noted in addition to the duration of infertility, because longer intervals since last impregnation may be associated with an increased chance of non-congenital disorders being the diagnosis.

PREVIOUS INVESTIGATIONS AND/OR TREATMENT FOR INFERTILITY

Information about previous investigations is important as this may save the need for repeat investigations. Details on previous treatments should be noted with information on whether the treatment was prescribed and taken correctly and the results.

2.3 **HISTORY OF DISEASES WITH POSSIBLE ADVERSE EFFECT ON FERTILITY**

The following systemic diseases have been reported to influence fertility:

Diabetes mellitus and neurological disease may cause erectile impotence and disorders of ejaculation. In addition, both conditions may damage spermatogenesis and the function of the accessory sex glands (Sexton & Jarow, 1997; Padron et al., 1997; Colpi et al., 1987).

Tuberculosis may cause epididymitis and prostatitis associated with impairment of sperm transport. Chronic respiratory tract disease includes chronic sinusitis, chronic bronchitis, and bronchiectasis. These conditions are sometimes associated with disorders of the sperm flagellum, such as in the immotile cilia syndrome, or with secretory disturbance in the epididymis with obstructive azoospermia. The latter problem may also occur in men with cystic fibrosis; these men also have an increased incidence of dysgenesis or absence of the vas deferens based on the same genetic defect (see Examination of the vasa deferentia, p. 22).

Other non-genital diseases which have been associated with infertility should also be recorded (see Table 2.2).

Orchitis associated with infectious parotitis (mumps) is recorded as a possible cause of acquired testicular damage rather than as a systemic disease.

Note that excessive alcohol consumption, whilst causing systemic disease in multiple organs including the liver and probably indirectly the testis, should be recorded separately.

2.3.1 **Fever**

A fever exceeding 38.5 °C may suppress spermatogenesis for a period of up to 6 months (World Health Organization, 1987). Recent data suggest that fever may also be associated with

Table 2.2. *Diseases associated with male infertility*

Disease	Mechanism
Congenital disorders	
Genetic disorders	
Kartagener's syndrome	Immotile sperm
Cystic fibrosis	Associated with agenesis of vas deferens and also with secretory disturbance in epididymis
Androgen receptor deficiency	Lack of development of genitalia
Prune belly syndrome	Testicular maldescent
Coeliac disease	Testicular damage
Testicular maldescent	Testicular damage
Von-Hippel–Lindau syndrome	Cystadenoma of epididymis
Acquired disorders	
Infections	
Infectious parotitis (mumps)	Orchitis
Tuberculosis	Obstruction and orchitis
Bilharziasis	Obstruction
Gonorrhoea	Obstruction (and orchitis)
Chlamydial epididymitis	Obstruction
Filariasis	Obstruction
Typhoid	Orchitis
Influenza	Orchitis
Undulant fever (Brucellosis)	Orchitis
Syphilis	Orchitis
Pemphigus foliaceus in South America	Azoospermia (? obstruction)
Endocrine disease	
Thyrotoxicosis	Hormonal abnormality
Diabetes mellitus	Testicular failure and ejaculatory disturbance
Hepatic failure	Hormonal abnormality
Renal failure	Testicular failure and loss of libido
Secondary testicular failure	Pituitary failure; usually there will also be androgen deficiency
Chromophobe adenoma	
Astrocytoma	
Hamartoma	
Teratoma	
Sarcoidosis	
Neurological disease	
Paraplegia	Erectile impotence and disorders of ejaculation; damage to spermatogenesis; damage to accessory sex glands
Chronic respiratory tract disease	
Bronchiectasis	May be associated with abnormal sperm cilia in the
Chronic sinusitis	immotile cilia syndrome, situs inversus or secretory
Chronic bronchitis	disturbance in the epididymis such as in Young's syndrome

Source: Adapted from Hargreave, 1994.

sperm DNA damage. Details should be recorded of the disease or condition causing the hyperthermia, its duration and treatment. It is not known, for example, whether the deleterious influence of an attack of influenza may be less than that following a severe malarial episode.

2.3.2 Medical interventions

Certain medical treatments may cause temporary or permanent damage to spermatogenesis.

Some of the therapeutic drugs which may interfere with fertility are listed in Table 2.3. If there is a history of medication with one of these drugs, consideration needs to be given as to whether it is safe to stop the drug or whether there are any alternative preparations without deleterious effects on sexual function or semen quality (e.g. substitution of mesalazine instead of sulphasalazine in men with chronic inflammatory disease of the intestine such as Crohn's disease and ulcerative colitis) (Forman et al., 1996).

Cancer therapy
Testicular cancer, Hodgkin's disease, non-Hodgkin lymphomas and leukaemia may affect young people, and the disease or its treatment may have deleterious effects on fertility. Irradiation in the genital region will most probably cause irreversible arrest of spermatogenesis with subsequent sterility. Among cancer chemotherapy, the alkylating agents usually cause irreversible damage. In all cases, semen cryopreservation should be offered prior to treatment and not during treatment (Meistrich, 1993).

2.3.3 History of surgery

There may be temporary depression of fertility which may last for 3 to 6 months after any surgical procedure, particularly after general anaesthesia has been administered. The following surgical procedures may influence fertility directly.

Testicular biopsy may result in a temporary suppression of spermatogenesis.

Treatment of urethral valves in infancy, prostatectomy or bladder neck incision for outflow obstruction may result in retrograde ejaculation.

Urinary catheterization may be complicated by urinary tract infection (see below) or by urethral stricture.

Table 2.3. *Some therapeutic drugs which may have side effects of interference with male fertility*

Name of drug	Relevance to male fertility
Cancer chemotherapy	See text.
Hormone treatments	High dose corticosteroids, androgens and antiandrogens, progestogens, estrogens and LHRH (GnRH) (super)agonists or antagonists. For example, anabolic steroids may be taken by some athletes and young men who are weight training. These steroids can interfere with feedback to the pituitary causing a reduction in gonadotrophin secretion and testicular atrophy which usually is reversible.
Cimetidine	May competitively inhibit androgen effect on the receptor.
Sulphasalazine	Causes impairment of sperm quality by direct toxicity.
Spironolactone	May antagonize action of androgens in some tissues.
Nitrofurantoin	May cause impairment of sperm quality by direct toxicity.
Niridazole	Is an antischistosomal agent which inhibits spermatogenesis in the gonads of the schistosome, and may also cause a temporary depression of fertility in man.
Colchicine	Has been reported to cause depression of fertility by direct toxicity on spermatogenesis.

Note:
Other drugs that may interfere with reproductive function include some antihypertensives and tranquillizers which interfere with erectile potency or ejaculation (for a more comprehensive list of drugs, see Forman et al., 1996).

Urethral stricture repair may result in pooling of ejaculate material in a flaccid segment of the urethra and its contamination with urine. There may be ejaculatory disturbance after reconstructive surgery for hypospadias, epispadias and vesicular exstrophy.

Hernia repair (particularly in young children) may result in damage to the vas deferens with partial or complete obstruction, or an immunological reaction with production of antisperm antibodies. This may also occur after hydrocelectomy or any other genital or inguinal surgery.

Vasectomy is the most common cause of surgical obstruction and also results in production of antisperm antibodies. These antibodies persist after the repair operation and may hinder natural conception, even if obstruction has been relieved correctly.

Lumbar sympathectomy may occur after lymphadenectomy or major retroperitoneal surgery and results in ejaculatory disturbance, both retrograde ejaculation and anejaculation.

Note should be made of the date of the operation and of any postoperative complications. Operations for varicocele, testicular torsion or testicular maldescent are recorded separately. Other operations should be noted if the investigator suspects relevance to infertility.

2.3.4 Urinary tract infection

The patient should be questioned about any history of dysuria, urethral discharge, pyuria, haematuria, frequency of micturition or other urinary symptoms. The number of occurrences and the treatment should be recorded. Inadequate treatment or recurrent episodes may be associated with accessory gland infection and poor semen quality.

2.3.5 Sexually transmitted disease

Information should be collected about *Syphilis*, gonorrhoea and *Chlamydia trachomatis* infection or other sexually transmitted diseases, such as *Lymphogranuloma venereum*, mycoplasma infection or non-specific urethritis. The number of episodes, the number of months since the last episode and treatment should be recorded. NB These patients are more likely to contract HIV infection.

There is increasing awareness that *Chlamydia trachomatis* infection is a common cause of epididymitis. The organism is difficult to detect, and almost certainly the true incidence has been underreported because of difficulties with laboratory identification techniques.

Recent studies suggest that infertile men may have a high incidence of herpes simplex and human papilloma virus DNA positivity in their semen (el-Borai et al., 1997; Lai et al., 1997) and that the presence of human papilloma virus in semen may have an effect on sperm motility. Further studies are needed to assess the role of these viruses in male infertility.

2.3.6 Epididymitis

Most patients are unable to distinguish between epididymo-orchitis and chronic epididymitis. The clinician should try to distinguish between the two, namely, acute generalized and severe scrotal pain suggestive of epididymo-orchitis and recurrent well localized pain or discomfort (which may however change localization) suggestive of chronic epididymitis.

2.4 PATHOLOGY POSSIBLY CAUSING TESTICULAR DAMAGE

2.4.1 Mumps orchitis

The classical orchitis is associated with infectious parotitis (mumps), but orchitis is seen with other viral infections, e.g. coxsackie or herpes. Following an attack of mumps orchitis, the recovery of fertility is variable; some men remain sterile and in other cases the time to recovery of sperm production may take as long as 2 years.

Mumps occurring before puberty and mumps not accompanied by orchitis do not interfere with fertility and need not be recorded.

2.4.2 Testicular injury

Testicular trauma as a cause of infertility is rare. A history of minor scrotal injury is common but it is improbable that this is important in producing fertility problems. Injury should be recorded if it was accompanied by signs of tissue damage such as scrotal haematoma, haematospermia or haematuria. Subsequent testicular atrophy is a strong indication of the relevance of the traumatic incident. Severe injury, even when unilateral, may be important as it may cause disruption of the blood–testis barrier and initiate antisperm antibody production.

2.4.3 Testicular torsion

Testicular torsion is a relatively infrequent cause of infertility. Later fertility problems may be prevented by early treatment (operation within 6 hours of onset of symptoms). Fixation of the contralateral testis is also indicated.

The diagnosis should always be suspected in prepubertal boys and in adolescents who develop acute painful swelling in the scrotum.

2.4.4 History of varicocele

A history of varicocele requires details about the mode of treatment, including the surgical technique or the method of embolization, possible complications and the age at which treatment was performed. Also, any investigations that were performed to evaluate the technical success of the treatment should be recorded. A previous varicocele should not be regarded as the cause of abnormal semen quality if this persists for two or more years following effective treatment of the varicocele (defined as absence of venous reflux after treatment).

2.4.5 Testicular maldescent

The patient should be asked whether both testes have always been in the scrotum. If they have not, details should be recorded about the age, mode and result of treatment, and possible complications. Untreated bilaterally undescended testes are associated with sterility, and impairment in fertility is common in untreated or even treated unilateral cases. Treatment (before puberty) may sometimes prevent later infertility.

There is a risk of malignant change in testicular maldescent and this is particularly true in intraabdominal testes (Batata et al., 1980; Campbell, 1959). The increased risk may persist after the testis has been placed in the scrotum and it is also present in the contralateral testis of patients with unilateral cryptorchidism. Management should take this into account.

Testes may be retractile, ectopic or have arrested descent (see Physical examination p. 18).

2.5 OTHER FACTORS WITH POSSIBLE ADVERSE EFFECT ON FERTILITY

Certain environmental, occupational and lifestyle factors are suspected to interfere with normal spermatogenesis.

Relatively little is known about the working environment and its possible effects on male infertility. Excessively hot environments may depress spermatogenesis. Also, some studies suggest that exposure of the testis to elevated temperature during bathing or prolonged driving may temporarily suppress spermatogenesis (Mieusset & Bujan, 1995; Thonneau & Mieusset, 1997). Chronic exposure to heavy metals, e.g. lead, cadmium and mercury or other substances, e.g. pesticides, herbicides, carbon disulphide may also reduce fertility. Some authors are convinced that exposure to substances with hormone disrupting properties such as the pseudo-oestrogens DDT, polychlorinated biphenyls, Bisphenol A, alkyl phenols, phthalates or antiandrogens may cause malformations of the genital tract, reduce sperm production and impair spermatogenesis (Sharpe & Skakkebaek, 1993).

Chronic excessive alcohol consumption may interfere with spermatogenesis and also reduce sexual function through inhibition of testosterone biosynthesis. These effects are prominent if alcohol abuse occurs on an almost daily basis and exceeds approximately six units per day.

Recent literature meta-analyses indicate tobacco smoking is associated with modest reductions in semen quality, increased oxidative damage to the sperm DNA, and alterations in serum hormone levels. It has been reported that excessive tobacco smoking can enhance the deleterious effects of genital diseases (e.g. varicocele) (Klaiber et al., 1987; Mahmoud et al., 1998c) or other environmental factors on spermatogenesis. Also, men who smoke have a higher number of white blood cells in semen (Close et al., 1990), an increased risk of urethritis (Martin-Boyce et al., 1977) and impaired secretory functions of male accessory sex glands (Pakrashi & Chatterjee, 1995).

There have been reports that marihuana smoking is associated with reduction in fertility. Men who become addicted to opiate drugs often have multiple episodes of septicaemia and poor general health, and it is difficult to know if any damage to fertility is a direct result of the drug or of self-neglect.

The misuse of anabolic steroids, e.g. for body-building may suppress spermatogenesis.

2.5.1 Sexual and ejaculatory function

Difficulties with sexual intercourse or ejaculation causing infertility are identified in about 2% of couples. They may be associated with overt disease such as paraplegia or other acquired neurological disorders.

These problems are not always evident from history-taking and may only be detected during investigations because the man is unable or unwilling to provide a semen sample for analysis, or the wife is found to have an intact hymen, or there may be no spermatozoa seen in a postcoital test.

If the average frequency of vaginal intercourse is twice or less per month, it should be recorded as inadequate. This may be an aetiological factor in the couple's infertility. Some couples, however, concentrate on a recognized fertile period, and understanding of the assessment of the timing of ovulation may be consistent with a low frequency of intercourse. In this situation the low frequency may be considered adequate.

For the purpose of the investigation of infertility, penile erection is considered adequate if it is sufficient to permit vaginal intercourse. Erectile impotence or penile deformity requires additional investigations to identify its possible aetiological mechanism(s).

Ejaculation should occur intravaginally to be considered as adequate. Anejaculation, extreme forms of ejaculation praecox (taking place before intromission), extravaginal ejaculation, e.g. associated with extreme hypospadias, and retrograde ejaculation should be recorded as inadequate. Similar to men with erectile impotence, patients with ejaculatory disturbances need further investigations to detect a possible cause.

Psychological problems as the main cause of infertility are uncommon. However, psychological problems sometimes occur after prolonged infertility investigations and may result in sexual or ejaculatory dysfunction. An important aspect of management of the couple with a fertility problem is counselling.

3 Clinical assessment of male fertility

3.1 **PHYSICAL EXAMINATION**

The man should be examined in a warm room (20–22 °C) in privacy. It is recommended that the subject is completely undressed during the general physical examination.

3.1.1 General examination

A general physical examination should be performed to detect abnormalities relevant to fertility.

Measurement of height, weight and blood pressure may give information about systemic disease. Gross overweight (a body mass index of ≥ 30 kg/m^2) has been associated with reduced testicular volume, suggesting impairment of spermatogenesis (World Health Organization, 1987).

In Klinefelter syndrome there is often disproportionately long limb length in relation to trunk length. However, the absence of this physical sign does not exclude the diagnosis.

Signs of hypoandrogenism include poor expression of secondary sex characteristics. The body hair distribution gives an indication of androgen production, and scanty pubic hair may suggest hypoandrogenism. This may be backed up by questions about the frequency of shaving. Depending on the patient's ethnic origin, infrequent shaving may indicate relatively low androgen production. Any abnormality of secondary sexual development should be staged according to the pubertal development scale of Tanner (1962) (Appendix II.1).

3.1.2 Gynaecomastia

The breasts should be inspected and palpated for the presence or absence of glandular tissue. This is best done with the patient's hands placed behind his head to extend the pectoral muscles.

The degree of gynaecomastia is classified into stages as described by Tanner (see Appendix II.2). Mild gynaecomastia is commonly seen in pubertal boys without any obvious hormonal abnormality and may sometimes persist after puberty. It is classically described as part of the Klinefelter syndrome. Gynaecomastia may also result from exposure to endogenous or exogenous oestrogens or medication such as digitalis, spironolactone, etc. An oestrogen-secreting tumour of the adrenal gland or the testis is another rare cause.

3.1.3 Examination of the penis

The penis should be inspected and palpated to detect hypospadias, surgical or traumatic scars, induration plaques or other pathology. The foreskin should be retracted, when any phimosis will become apparent. The external urethral meatus should be identified. Hypospadias, epispadias, and other penile deformities are only relevant to infertility if they prevent intercourse or when semen is delivered outside of the vagina. Scars related to previous surgery may be indicative of urethral strictures, which itself may result in ejaculatory dysfunction.

A common complaint is that the size of the penis is perceived as too small for satisfactory intercourse. In fact, micropenis is very rare (it may occur as part of 5-α-reductase deficiency syndrome; Imperato-MacGinley et al., 1974) and is almost never the cause of infertility. Usually, reassurance from the examining doctor is all that is required.

Any ulceration or urethral discharge should be noted and, if present, further investigations should be undertaken to identify the sexually transmitted disease.

3.1.4 Examination of the testes

The site of the testes is best determined with the man standing. The testes should both be palpable and low in the scrotum.

Any abnormality in the site of the testes should be categorized as follows.

Retractile testes

This condition must be differentiated from maldescent. The testes lie normally in the scrotum but, as the cremasteric reflexes develop, each may retract to the external inguinal ring. This reflex is most marked in 5- and 6-year-olds but can be prominent in adults. The role of retractile testes as a cause of infertility is still a matter of debate. This condition must not be recorded as undescended testes.

Ectopic testes

Testes are considered ectopic when there is deviation from the normal path of descent. The commonest type of ectopic testis lies in the superficial inguinal pouch. Rarely, they may be found in other sites, e.g. femoral canal, pubic region or in the opposite side of the scrotum.

Incomplete descent

The testes may arrest at any point on the normal pathway of descent between the posterior abdominal wall and the external inguinal ring. The testis may be:

- high in the scrotum, i.e. at the scrotal neck;
- inguinal: lying within the inguinal canal;
- impalpable.

Impalpable testes may be either located in the inguinal canal or intraabdominally. Complete absence of the testes is rare but can be distinguished from intraabdominal testes by the lack of increase in serum testosterone levels after human chorionic gonadotrophin stimulation.

The position and axis of the testes should be noted with the man standing. Normally, the testis lies in the scrotum vertically with the epididymis behind or median. The testes may retract into the inguinal canal and this may be a problem, particularly if it occurs during sexual intercourse and causes pain. However, this probably has no relevance to fertility. Horizontally lying testes are thought to be more liable to torsion (Williamson, 1976). If such a patient gives a history of intermittent pain, and particularly if testicular volume is reduced or sperm concentration is low, testicular fixation should be considered.

Estimation of testicular volume is performed with the patient in recumbent position because of the risk of syncope. The scrotal skin is stretched over the testis, the contours of which are isolated from the epididymis (Fig. 3.1). The volume of each testis is compared with the corresponding ovoid of the Prader orchio-

Fig. 3.1. Measurement of testicular volume by Prader orchiometer.

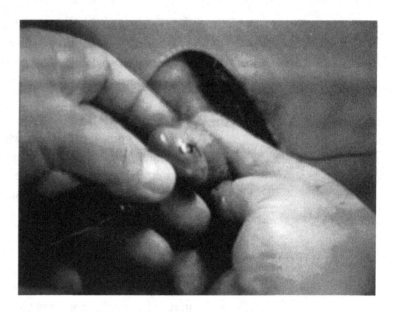

meter. Other methods for the estimation of testicular volume have been recommended including ultrasonography, the 'punch through' orchiometer (Takihara et al., 1983) and calipers. The normal size may relate to ethnic group, but mostly depends on stature. Most of the volume is accounted for by the seminiferous tubule mass. There is a strong correlation between the total testicular volume, which is the sum of the left and right testes, and the total number of spermatozoa (sperm count) per ejaculate (Fig. 3.2) (World Health Organization, 1987).

Small-sized testes may indicate insufficiency of the seminiferous epithelium. For Caucasian men this is a size of less than 15 ml, but there are racial differences in testicular volume (Diamond, 1986). Small testes, usually no more than 3 ml, in volume, are found in men with Klinefelter syndrome. Patients with hypogonadotrophic hypogonadism also have small testes, but the size usually is between 5 and 12 ml. A normal testicular volume in a man with azoospermia may indicate obstruction. An unduly large and asymmetrical testis may indicate testicular tumour. Symmetrical large testes, also called macro-orchia (a testis volume of more than 35 ml each) (World Health Organization, 1987), is an occasional normal finding or it may be a characteristic of the fragile X syndrome (Hagerman et al., 1991). In case of large testicular volume, echography (ultrasonography examination) of the scrotal contents is mandatory to

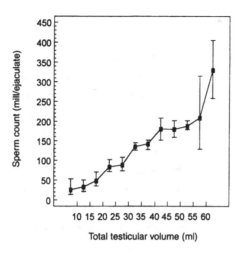

Fig. 3.2. Correlation between the total testicular volume, which is the sum of the left and the right side added, and the total number of spermatozoa (sperm count) per ejaculate in cases without obstruction (WHO, 1987).

exclude the presence of a testicular tumour. False estimation of testicular volume may occur if there is hydrocele.

Testicular consistency should be estimated by gentle pressure. The normal consistency is rubbery. Soft testes are nearly always associated with impaired spermatogenesis. Occasionally, patients are found with a hard testis of normal or large volume, and a testicular tumour may be present. If testes are small and hard, Klinefelter syndrome is suspected, whereas small and soft testes are commonly found in men with hypogonadotropic hypogonadism.

3.1.5 Examination of the epididymides

The normal epididymis is barely palpable, has a regular outline and soft consistency. Gentle palpation does not cause pain. Painful nodules may indicate epididymitis or sperm granulomata. Those in the caput epididymidis suggest infection by *Chlamydia trachomatis*. Painful swelling and/or nodularity of the caudal region may indicate either gonococcal infection, or inflammation or infection with common urinary pathogens such as *E. coli*, *Proteus* or *Klebsiella* species. Sperm granulomata after previous vasectomy are usually also found in the caudal region. Cystic deformities may, or may not, be relevant to any obstruction. The epididymis may be distended in cases with obstructive azoospermia.

During epididymal palpation the following points should be noted.

- Is the epididymis palpable?
- Is the anatomical relationship to the testis normal, i.e. does the epididymis lie close to the testis; above, behind and below the testis? Anatomical variations may occur, e.g. the epididymis may lie anterior to the testis (may be injured during surgical procedures, e.g. testicular biopsy).
- Are there any cysts, indurated or nodular areas, or any other abnormalities and, if yes, are these abnormal areas located in the head, body or tail?
- Does gentle palpation cause pain?

3.1.6 Examination of the vasa deferentia

Both vasa deferentia should be palpated. Normally, the vas is felt as a thin, firm, cord-like structure passing between the examining fingers. However, clinicians will sometimes miss bilateral absence of the vasa and it is worth reexamining all men with azoospermia, particularly if the testicular volume is normal and the ejaculate has a low volume and acidic pH. Congenital agenesis of the vasa deferentia, whether complete or not, is associated with homo- or heterozygous defects of the cystic fibrosis transmembrane conductance regulator gene, and may be associated with mild or moderate clinical stigmata of cystic fibrosis. Unilateral absence is much rarer and may also be associated with an absence of the kidney on the same side. Azoospermic patients with ejaculates of small volume and low pH should also be tested for cystic fibrosis even if the vasa are palpable, for sometimes only the abdominal section of the vas is absent.

If the vas is present, a note should be made of whether it is normal, thickened, nodular or painful upon pressure as this may indicate inflammation.

3.1.7 Scrotal swelling

Fig. 3.3 shows a scheme for the clinical diagnosis of scrotal swellings. If in doubt, the best additional test is ultrasonography examination.

Congenital hernia with a patent processus vaginalis may be relevant, as this may be associated with testicular maldescent. Any hernia, when associated with reduced testicular volume and abnormal semen quality, may be relevant to infertility.

Fig. 3.3. Scheme for the clinical diagnosis for scrotal swellings.

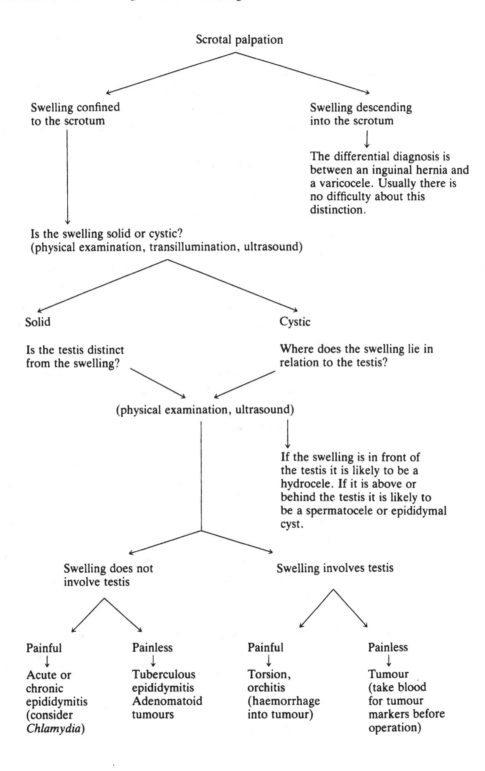

A large hydrocele may interfere with fertility but there is controversy about this. It must be remembered that sometimes the hydrocele is a reaction to underlying testicular tumour.

3.1.8 Varicocele

The examination room should be about 20 to 22 °C. The patient should stand undressed for 5 minutes before being examined. At lower temperature the scrotum may retract, making palpation difficult. The patient should be standing up while the scrotum is inspected and palpated. Varicoceles can be categorized into:

- grade III, when the distended venous plexus bulges visibly through the scrotal skin and is easily palpable;
- grade II, when intrascrotal venous distention is easily palpable but not visible;
- grade I, when there is no visible or palpable distention except when the man performs the Valsalva manoeuvre;
- subclinical, when there is no clinical varicocele, but an abnormality is present upon scrotal thermography or Doppler ultrasonography.

The diagnosis of grade I and subclinical varicocele should be confirmed by additional investigations (p. 31).

3.1.9 Inguinal examination

Care should be taken to examine for inguinal scars as this may indicate surgery for previous testicular maldescent, or there may have been injury to the vas deferens during operation for hernia. Such scars may be difficult to see as they are often covered by pubic hair. Scars in the inguinal area may also indicate past or current infection with tuberculosis or *Lymphogranuloma venereum*. The presence of pathological enlargement of inguinal lymph nodes or inguinal hernia should be recorded.

3.1.10 Examination of the prostate gland and seminal vesicles

This may be omitted if there is no history, physical signs or indication from urine or semen analysis that the patient may have any disease of the accessory sex glands.

Examination of the prostate gland is by rectal examination preferentially with the man in the knee–elbow position.

Palpation should be performed from cranial to the caudal part of the prostate and from lateral to medial. The normal prostate is soft, regular and not painful on slight pressure. The central groove should be easily identified. Soft swelling which is tender may indicate inflammation. Pain is often felt as a burning sensation irradiating along the penile urethra. This has to be distinguished from the general unpleasant sensation that the patient will usually describe. Stony hardness of the prostate may indicate malignant growth but this is very uncommon in men consulting with infertility.

The seminal vesicles are not normally palpable. If they are palpable and/or painful upon pressure this usually indicates inflammation. In general, seminal vesiculitis is accompanied by prostatitis. Some men with characteristics of obstructive azoospermia have cystic deformities of the seminal vesicles, others may have agenesis which is associated with congenital agenesis of the vasa deferentia. Abnormalities of the prostate and/or seminal vesicles are best detected by echography, preferably using a rectal probe.

3.2   LABORATORY INVESTIGATIONS

3.2.1   Semen analysis

In the investigation of an infertile couple, at least one semen analysis is always mandatory, even if the postcoital test appears to be normal. Semen analysis includes the assessment of the characteristics of spermatozoa and of seminal plasma, and must be performed using standardized methods at least equivalent to the minimum standards described in the *WHO Laboratory Manual for the Examination of Human Semen and Sperm–Cervical Mucus Interaction* (CUP, 4th edn, 1999). Semen samples could transmit HIV and other infections. Therefore, suitable precautions should be taken when handling semen samples.

Semen classification uses the following nomenclature.

Normozoospermia: normal ejaculate as defined by the reference values (see Appendix III).
Oligozoospermia: less than the reference value for sperm concentration.
Asthenozoospermia: less than the reference value for motility.
Teratozoospermia: less than the reference value for morphology.

Oligoasthenoterato-zoospermia: signifies disturbance of all three variables (combination of only two prefixes may also be used).

Cryptozoospermia: no spermatozoa observed in the fresh sample but a few spermatozoa are recovered in the sediment after centrifugation.

Azoospermia: no spermatozoa in the ejaculate (confirmed after centrifugation).

Aspermia: no ejaculate.

Errors in semen sample collection (e.g. loss of a part of the sample, the use of condoms containing a spermicide) and transport (i.e. exposure of the sample to extremes of temperature, or a delay in semen analysis more than 2 hours after ejaculation) and contamination of the sample with urine, water, soap, etc., should be excluded since they may lead to false conclusions regarding semen quality (for further details see *WHO Laboratory Manual for the Examination of Human Semen and Sperm–Cervical Mucus Interaction,* CUP, 4th edn, 1999).

If the first semen analysis is normal, there is usually no need for a repeat analysis. The results of semen analysis should be interpreted in conjunction with the findings at clinical examination. There is no need to repeat semen analysis in a case of azoospermia and bilateral agenesis of the vas deferens. In all other circumstances with abnormal semen classification, a repeat analysis must be performed. If the result of the second analysis is remarkably different from that of the first analysis, additional semen samples may be needed at a longer time interval before any decision is taken as to the management of the male (see also Interpretation of the results of semen analysis, p. 37).

3.2.2 Other laboratory investigations

3.2.2.1 *Tests on blood and serum*

Screening blood analysis may be indicated to detect certain systemic diseases with possible influence on fertility. It may include estimation of haemoglobin concentration, red and white blood cell count, sedimentation rate, tests of renal and hepatic function, serum iron concentration, and other tests depending on the findings of physical examination or history taking and on the regional situation.

Specific testing for immunoglobulins against *Chlamydia trachomatis* in serum has no diagnostic relevance for acute chlamydial infection (see below and p. 52).

Specific testing for antibodies against HIV may be elective or mandatory depending on the prevalence of HIV in the general population and man's history and physical examination. Before testing the patient for HIV, consent must be obtained and the patient should be counselled.

Several tests are often used for the detection and titration of antisperm antibodies in serum but the indications and the interpretation of these tests are controversial. Among these the indirect mixed antiglobulin reaction using coated latex particles and the indirect Immunobead test are most suitable (although the sensitivity and specificity of the latter has been reported as less good; Andreou et al., 1995).

3.2.2.2   *Tests on urine*

It is good clinical practice to perform routine urine analysis.

For the diagnosis of *Chlamydia trachomatis* infection, a first-voided urine (FVU) sample is an important alternative procedure for specimen collection and obviates the need for urethral swabbing, which is often unacceptable in the asymptomatic subject. The urine specimen can be tested for *Chlamydia trachomatis* by DNA amplification techniques such as polymerase chain reaction (PCR) or ligase chain reaction (LCR). These techniques may offer better opportunities to detect *Chlamydia* infection. ELISA *Chlamydia* antigen detection kits can also be employed on FVU specimens, but are less sensitive than PCR or LCR, and positive tests require confirmation by a DNA amplification technique.

Postorgasm urine

In men with aspermia or with low ejaculate volume, one should consider the possibility of (partial) retrograde ejaculation which is a form of ejaculatory inadequacy. The patient should be asked to have an orgasm during either intercourse or masturbation and then to void urine. Cloudy appearance of the urine with the presence of a total number of spermatozoa in urine equal to, or exceeding, the number of spermatozoa in semen strongly supports the diagnosis of retrograde ejaculation.

Urine collected after prostatic massage

The collection of multiple aliquots of urine may be performed for the diagnosis and localization of male accessory gland infection: this includes the collection of the urethral urine, midstream urine and postmassage urine (Maers & Stamey, 1968).

3.2.2.3 Prostatic expressed fluid

Although examination of prostatic expressed fluid is common practice, it is not recommended because it is unpleasant to the patient and criteria for interpretation are poorly defined.

3.2.2.4 Hormone determinations

Hormone determinations are rarely needed for diagnostic classification and should be performed only when indicated (see below). A recent study of infertile men indicated that screening of men with a sperm concentration of less than 10 million/ml with serum testosterone and follicle stimulating hormone (FSH) alone will detect the vast majority of clinically significant endocrine abnormalities (Sigman & Jarow, 1998). Determinations must use well-standardized techniques and be interpreted with reference to the assaying laboratory's normal range, as defined for normal adult men with proven fertility.

Measurement of serum follicle stimulating hormone (FSH) is performed to discriminate between hypergonadotropic and normo- or hypogonadotrophic hypogonadism. It is indicated in men with azoospermia. In the absence of other recognized causes of impaired spermatogenesis, a normal serum FSH concentration may suggest obstruction of sperm transport. However, maturation arrest during spermatogenesis cannot be ruled out in these cases.

If FSH concentration is elevated, this indicates a severe defect in spermatogenesis including Sertoli-cell only syndrome (germ cell aplasia) or maturation arrest at an early stage, e.g. with only spermatogonia or primary spermatocytes present. In some of these patients spermatogenic arrest may be limited to localized regions of the seminiferous tubules, with other tubules exhibiting full spermatogenesis. Therefore, FSH determination is not useful in predicting whether spermatozoa are present in the testis, e.g. for use in intracytoplasmic sperm injection (ICSI) (Tournaye et al., 1997c). In men with low or slightly reduced testicular volume and signs of hypoandrogenism, the presence of a high serum FSH level suggests severe primary testicular failure impairing both spermatogenesis and Leydig cell function. If serum FSH level in not elevated in such men, hypogonadism may be due to functional hypothalamo-pituitary failure or to a pituitary tumour.

For the purpose of diagnostic classification, there is no need to determine serum FSH in patients with a demonstrable cause of infertility and spermatozoa present in the ejaculate. FSH estimation may, however, give prognostic information, as men who have, for example, varicocele with oligozoospermia and highly elevated FSH have little chance of recovering normal fertility after varicocele repair. In general, assessment of serum FSH concentration is not informative in patients with sperm concentration over 5 million per ml and normal testicular volume.

The concentration of inhibin B in serum is a good marker of spermatogenesis (Pierik et al., 1998), and may be more reliable than FSH measurement to assess this. The combined measurement of inhibin B and FSH probably gives the best estimation of spermatogenesis (van Eckardstein et al., 1999) and may help in distinguishing between testicular and non-testicular causes of abnormal sperm concentration (Mahmoud et al., 1998a).

Serum luteinizing hormone (LH) need not be measured in routine male infertility investigation. Cases with hypogonadotrophic hypogonadism can be diagnosed on the basis of a low plasma testosterone concentration and a serum FSH which is normal or low. If clinical hypoandrogenism is of primary testicular origin, serum FSH will be elevated. Some authors have suggested that a high LH/testosterone ratio may indicate Leydig cell resistance and predicts poor fertility prognosis, but this needs confirmation. The finding of low testosterone without elevated LH may indicate suppression of the hypothalamo-pituitary function by exogenous substances with hormonal activity, such as anabolic steroids or pseudo-oestrogens.

Plasma testosterone concentration needs to be measured in men with clinical signs of hypoandrogenism and in whom FSH is not elevated. In these cases, a low testosterone concentration indicates hypogonadotrophic hypogonadism of either pituitary or hypothalamic origin. In men with clinical signs of hypoandrogenism but elevated FSH concentration, testosterone measurement may be useful for clinical management with respect to androgen supplementation, but it is not needed for diagnostic classification. Testosterone measurement is also indicated in men with sexual dysfunction, as this may be associated with low androgen production.

Prolactin measurement is performed in men with sexual dysfunction, including decreased libido or inadequate penile erection, or with signs of hypoandrogenism, low testosterone concentration with the FSH not elevated. In all patients with an elevated prolactin, a repeat determination is mandatory. Stress, even the minor stress of venepuncture, may temporarily increase serum prolactin level.

If prolactin values remain elevated, the patient should be questioned about intake of tranquillizers, sulpiride, and other medication which may increase prolactin concentration. Also, thyroid function must be assessed, since hyperprolactinaemia may be associated with hypothyroidism. In cases with otherwise unexplained repeatedly elevated prolactin concentrations, imaging of the hypothalamo-pituitary region is indicated to detect a possible tumour. This may be a prolactinoma, or a tumour of the hypothalamic region, such as a craniopharyngioma, or a tumour causing compression of the pituitary stalk. In some cases hyperprolactinaemia is caused by pituitary stalk disruption, which may be accompanied by hypogonadotrophic hypogonadism.

Other steroids and hormones

Assessment of androgen precursors of adrenal or testicular origin, or androgen metabolites such as 5α-dihydrotestosterone, 5α-3α-androstanediol, or oestradiol is not needed for diagnostic classification. Some laboratories may perform these measurements for experimental reasons, but their clinical meaning is questionable.

Measurement of oestradiol may be indicated in some men with gynaecomastia, which may be due to adrenal or testicular tumours, and thyroid stimulating hormone assessment should be performed in men with suspected thyroid dysfunction.

3.2.2.5   *Chromosome and genetic analysis*

All infertile men with a sperm concentration below 5 to 10 million/ml should be screened for numerical and structural abnormalities of sex chromosomes and autosomes (Yoshida et al., 1996).

Y chromosome microdeletions in patients with poor sperm quality, who will be treated by ICSI, is under investigation because of the concern over transferring these microdeletions to the male offspring (see Notes on assisted reproduction, p. 59; Kent-First et al., 1996).

Testing both partners for cystic fibrosis gene mutations should be performed routinely in all patients with unilateral or bilateral absence of the vas deferens, other abnormalities of the vasa and/or abnormalities of the seminal vesicles on rectal ultrasonography, and in all azoospermic patients with ejaculates of small volume and low pH. A recent study suggested that these mutations also are more common in infertile men with poor semen quality and without absent vas deferens compared to the general population (van der Ven et al., 1996), although others were unable to confirm this finding (Tuerlings et al., 1998; Tournaye et al., 1997a). Therefore, analysis of a larger cohort may still be necessary to prove or disprove this association (Tuerlings et al., 1998).

Fluorescent in situ hybridization (FISH) and other tests of the genetic material of spermatozoa are presently under investigation and are not currently a routine investigation, but they may be useful for the diagnosis of chromosomal aneuploidy and for the evaluation of risk for the offspring (Moosani et al., 1995; Mercier & Bresson, 1997).

3.3   ADDITIONAL TECHNICAL INVESTIGATIONS

3.3.1   Scrotal thermography

In order to detect or confirm possible subclinical or grade I varicocele, respectively (see p. 24), scrotal thermography should be performed in patients with abnormal semen analysis and in those who present with no clinical abnormalities upon urogenital examination or with asymmetrically reduced testicular volume or with grade I varicocele. The patient has to stand undressed for about 5 minutes in a room where the temperature does not exceed 22 °C, to permit equilibration of the temperature of the scrotal skin. With the patient standing, the investigator brings the scrotum forwards with both hands and applies a flexible strip containing thermosensitive liquid crystals. The crystals change colour reflecting the temperature of the underlying scrotal skin. If available, telethermography may also be used.

In a normal man, the temperature of the scrotal skin does usually not exceed 33 °C. In the case of retrograde filling of the intrascrotal pampiniform plexus, the temperature of the scrotal skin overlying this plexus will commonly be increased. This is detected by a change in colour of the liquid crystals, indicating a temperature of over 33 °C. Any clear asymmetrical or symmetrical temperature increase must be noted, and further investigations are indicated to confirm the presence of subclinical varicocele. False-positive thermographic findings may occur in case of increased scrotal temperature, due to scrotal skin disease or inflammatory process in the underlying structures, particularly the epididymis. In case of normal scrotal thermography the probability of a varicocele being present is small.

3.3.2   Doppler investigations

3.3.2.1   *Doppler ultrasonography*
In addition to, or as an alternative to thermography, particularly in cases with suspect thermographic findings, Doppler ultrasonography can be performed. The patient should be in a recumbent position. The testicular artery is located in the spermatic cord. The patient is requested to perform a Valsalva manoeuvre by blowing with his mouth open against his hand, without letting the air escape. During the Valsalva manoeuvre the pulsations of the testicular artery may decrease, but no reflux of blood should occur. After release of the Valsalva manoeuvre, an increased venous efflux may occur. In a typical case of varicocele, venous reflux will occur during the Valsalva manoeuvre, and intense venous efflux is recorded after relief of the manoeuvre.

Doppler ultrasonography requires adequate participation by the patient and much experience on the part of the investigator. False-positive findings are common due to misinterpretation of, for example, contraction–relaxation of the cremasteric muscles. False-negative findings may result from insufficient increase in the intrathoracic pressure during the Valsalva manoeuvre.

3.3.2.2   *Duplex Doppler*
Those clinics having access to a duplex or colour Doppler apparatus may use this technique. Some authors consider this technique to be the gold standard for diagnosis of venous reflux to the pampiniform plexus. However, the correct performance and interpretation of this technique requires adequate co-operation of the patient and sufficient experience and skill of the examiner. A study comparing the outcome of this technique with that of retrograde venography of the internal spermatic vein(s) indicates it to be a useful tool for the diagnosis of varicocele (Trum et al., 1996).

3.3.3   Other imaging techniques

3.3.3.1   *Ultrasonography (echography)*
Ultrasonographic examination may be useful for examination of the scrotum, testis and epididymis, but does require an appropriate probe (with a minimum of 7.5 MHz and preferably 10 MHz), and is also dependent on skilled interpretation. Ultrasonographic examination is indicated in cases suspected of testicular tumour (see Examination of the testes, p. 20). Ultrasonography of the accessory sex glands, the prostate and seminal vesicles (p. 24), is recommended in case of suspected agenesis of the vasa deferentia or infection/inflammation in male accessory gland.

3.3.3.2   *Imaging of the hypothalamo-pituitary region*
Imaging of the hypothalamo-pituitary region and assessment of the visual fields is required in patients with hyperprolactinaemia or gonadotrophin deficiency. In these men additional investigations may be performed, such as the GnRH test and other tests of hypothalamo-pituitary function.

3.3.4   Testicular biopsy

Previously, testicular biopsy was indicated, for the purposes of diagnostic classification, only in patients with unexplained azoospermia and normal testicular volume and a normal serum concentration of FSH.

The worldwide incidence of testicular germ-cell cancer has more than doubled over the past 40 years. The incidence is higher in Scandinavia, Germany and New Zeland in comparison with other countries (for review see Bosl & Motzer, 1997). Some men attending with infertility have predisposing causes of testicular malignancy such as testicular maldescent, and a tumour may be found during physical examination as a coincidental finding.

Testicular spermatozoa are now used for intracytoplasmic sperm injection (ICSI) during in vitro fertilization (IVF), and studies suggest an increased risk of testicular carcinoma in situ (CIS), which usually precedes most testicular tumours, in idiopathic azoospermia (Skakkebaek, 1978; West et al., 1985; Giwercman et al., 1993). Therefore, it is suggested that testicular tissue from men with idiopathic azoospermia undergoing ICSI should be evaluated histologically for CIS and CIS may be considered in other infertile men in countries where the incidence of testicular malignancy is high ($\geq 0.5\%$). The incidence required for 'screening' of the overall population should be $\geq 1\%$. However, in cases with infertility the incidence of CIS is higher compared to the overall population.

Except when testicular CIS is suspected, the biopsy should only be performed when adequate microsurgical techniques are available to treat possible obstruction of sperm transport, and when facilities are available to cryopreserve spermatozoa and/or part of the testicular tissue for further use in assisted reproduction. Some microsurgeons prefer that biopsies should be avoided for fear of compromising any microsurgical procedure. A wet preparation (Jow et al., 1993) is useful for immediate intraoperative identification of spermatozoa. Each Centre should make its own policy after consultation with the microsurgical team, and depending on the availability of adequate techniques of assisted reproduction.

For the detection of CIS, testicular tissues are preferably fixed in formaldehyde solution. On the other hand, testicular tissue for histological evaluation of spermatogenesis should not be fixed in formaldehyde solution, since this will make adequate histological and cytological evaluation impossible. The most commonly used histological fixatives of testicular tissue are Bouin's or Steive's solutions.

For the purpose of diagnostic classification, testicular histology should be categorized as:

- spermatozoa present in (some of) the seminiferous tubules: when a full spermatogenic complement is found in most (some) of the seminiferous tubules;
- spermatozoa absent: when spermatogenesis is incomplete in all seminiferous tubules due to germ cell arrest, also called maturation arrest, either at the spermatid, spermatocyte or spermatogonal level.

When Sertoli cell-only syndrome (also called germ-cell aplasia) or seminiferous tubule hyalinization is found histopathologically in cases with elevated serum FSH, assisted reproduction may not be formally impossible because sometimes some spermatogenesis may be found in isolated tubules (Tournaye et al., 1997c).

Immature testicular histology should not be found since these patients have small soft testes and other signs of hypogonadotrophic hypogonadism and therefore do not need testicular biopsy for the purpose of diagnostic classification.

4 Objective criteria for diagnostic categories in the standardized management of male infertility

Based on the working definitions described above, the procedures for the investigation and diagnosis have been validated, and a diagnostic pathway has been elaborated.

As indicated, two semen samples are analysed according to the procedures described in the *WHO Laboratory Manual for the Examination of Human Semen and Sperm–Cervical Mucus Interaction* (CUP, 4th edn 1999). Each semen sample is classified separately into one of the nine categories given below, and the highest ranking sample is used to determine the man's semen classification. It must be stressed that assessment of sperm motility and morphology has been found to be poorly standardized between different laboratories (Cooper et al., 1992; Dunphy et al., 1989; Neuwinger et al., 1990). Therefore, normal limits for those variables are not given, but reference values are suggested. Each laboratory must assess the lower limit of normality for these variables, and adhere to internal and external quality control schemes.

4.1 SEMEN CLASSIFICATION

Interpretation of the result of semen analysis

The degree of the couple's infertility is defined by the relative degree of the fertility impairment of both partners. It has been documented that suppressing sperm concentration below 3 million/ml has a contraceptive efficacy equivalent to a Pearl index of 1.4 (conceptions per 100 couple years) (World Health Organization, 1996). Furthermore, comparison of sperm characteristics of cohorts of fertile, subfertile and infertile men, and statistical analysis using receiver operating characterisitics curves, have permitted the definition of criterion and cut-off values (Comhaire et al., 1987; Ombelet et al., 1997b). Criterion values correspond to the values for sperm concentration, motility and morphology which have the highest power or accuracy in discriminating between two populations, e.g. fertile vs. subfertile, or subfertile vs. infertile. Criterion values are, in general, higher than the 'cut-off' values, which are accepted as the lower limit of 'normality', and are usually defined as the fifth percentile of sperm characteristics of the fertile population. Furthermore, and particularly in the subfertile group, the degree of sperm deficiency is correlated with the degree of subfertility, that is to say the fecundability (probability of conception per cycle of exposure) or the time to pregnancy (TTP). It is feasible to define, with acceptable accuracy, criterion and cut-off values for sperm concentration and for 'total sperm motility', because these variables can be measured with reasonable accuracy and reproducibility by most laboratories. Determining the criterion and cut-off values for the proportion of motility grade (a) or proportion of spermatozoa with 'ideal' morphology is more difficult in view of the interlaboratory variability and differences in criteria and test circumstances applied in different laboratories (see also Appendix III).

Antibody-coated spermatozoa
MAR or Immunobead test: $\geq 50\%$ of motile spermatozoa are antibody coated.

Normal semen: normal spermatozoa with normal seminal plasma
Semen variables as in reference values of semen variables (Appendix III)
and agglutination = no
and seminal plasma: appearance and consistency: both normal
and biochemistry: normal
and white blood cells: less than 1×10^6/ml
and culture: negative, i.e. less than 1000 bacteria (colony forming unit: 'CFU') per ml.

Normal spermatozoa with agglutination, or abnormal seminal plasma or white blood cells
Spermatozoa: as in reference values (Appendix III) and either of the following

Agglutination = yes

and/or Seminal plasma: one of the following is abnormal

Volume

or appearance and/or consistency

or pH,

or biochemistry,

or white blood cells (increased number)

or culture: positive, i.e. over 1000 CFU per ml.

Teratozoospermia

Spermatozoa: Concentration and motility: as in reference values (Appendix III)

and morphology: less than the reference value for morphology (or above the reference value for teratozoospermia index)

Asthenozoospermia

Spermatozoa: Concentration as in reference values (Appendix III)

and motility: less than the reference value for motility

Oligozoospermia

Spermatozoa: Concentration less than the reference value for concentration (Appendix III)

Cryptozoospermia:

Spermatozoa: No spermatozoa detected during routine semen analysis

and few spermatozoa are detected after centrifugation of semen specimen

Azoospermia

Spermatozoa: Concentration: $= 0.0 \times 10^6$/ml

and no spermatozoa are detected after centrifugation of semen specimen

Aspermia

Seminal plasma: Volume: $= 0.0$ ml

The overall semen classification is taken as the higher ranking classification of the two samples where 'antibody-coated spermatozoa' has the highest rank and 'aspermia' the lowest.

NB Some authors suggest that men who repeatedly have a normal semen volume and very high sperm concentration (>250 million/ml) should be classified as polyzoospermia. This has been reported in association with reduced fertility, but its relevance as a cause of infertility remains questionable (see p. 57).

4.2 **DIAGNOSTIC CATEGORIES AND MANAGEMENT**

On the basis of the man's semen classification, history and physical examination and additional diagnostic tests one of the diagnostic categories defined below is assigned according to the flowchart (see Appendix I). It is recommended that a complete diagnostic profile be reached for each individual patient by marking the logic on the flowchart. Several causal diagnoses may be present simultaneously. A suggested management strategy based on an extensive review of the literature is also given below.

A combination of male and female causes is detected in approximately one-quarter of couples with infertility. Hence, there is an approximately 50% probability of a female factor to be associated in case of male infertility. Such association may be coincidental or causal (e.g. an STD-induced pathology in both the male and female partners). In some infertile couples presenting initially with isolated male partner pathology, complementary pathology develops in the female during follow-up (e.g. ovulatory disturbance). This underscores the need for careful monitoring of both partners. Also, optimizing the female reproductive condition (e.g. by means of gonadotrophin support treatment) may increase the probability of conception.

In at least 25% of subfertile men more than one causal factor can be identified. Coincidence of factors may be fortuitous since certain pathologies are rather common, e.g. varicocele with congenital factor such as cryptorchidism or Y-chromosome gene deletion (which should be suspected in cases with small varicocele but reduced total testicular volume of <30 ml). Sometimes factors have been reported to present a causal relation, e.g. male accessory gland infection and immunological factor.

Recent studies suggest a multiplicative effect of different

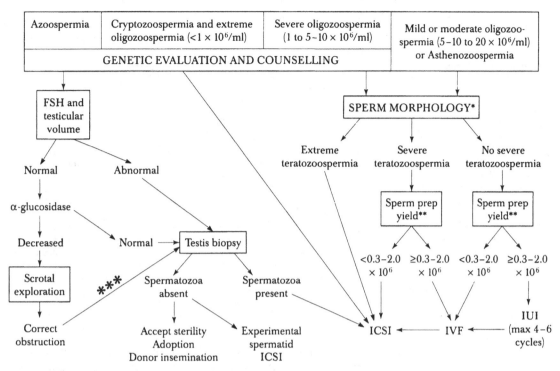

| Azoospermia | Cryptozoospermia and extreme oligozoospermia (<1 × 10⁶/ml) | Severe oligozoospermia (1 to 5–10 × 10⁶/ml) | Mild or moderate oligozoospermia (5–10 to 20 × 10⁶/ml) or Asthenozoospermia |

GENETIC EVALUATION AND COUNSELLING

FSH and testicular volume

Normal — Abnormal

α-glucosidase

Decreased — Normal → Testis biopsy

Scrotal exploration   ***

Correct obstruction

Spermatozoa absent

Accept sterility
Adoption
Donor insemination

Spermatozoa present

Experimental spermatid ICSI

SPERM MORPHOLOGY*

Extreme teratozoospermia

Severe teratozoospermia

No severe teratozoospermia

Sperm prep yield**

Sperm prep yield**

<0.3–2.0 × 10⁶   ≥0.3–2.0 × 10⁶   <0.3–2.0 × 10⁶   ≥0.3–2.0 × 10⁶

IUI (max 4–6 cycles)

ICSI ← IVF ←

Fig. 4.1. Management, general guidelines
* Sperm morphology is assessed as described in the *WHO Laboratory Manual* (CUP, 4th edn, 1999), providing the per cent normal forms and the Teratozoospermia Index (TZI). Management of men with teratozoospermia follows the general principles described in Appendix IV.
** Sperm preparation yield is defined as the number of progressively motile spermatozoa that may be recovered after processing an entire ejaculate from the man, see Appendix IV.
*** If available, epididymal spermatozoa can be aspirated for ICSI as part of the microepididymal sperm aspiration (MESA) procedure.

factors on sperm deterioration. This means that lifestyle, genital, and perhaps genetic causes may act in synergy, amplifying the unfavourable effect of each single factor. It seems that this synergism results from a common pathogenetic mechanism, namely oxidative damage induced by increased generation of reactive oxygen species and/or decreased antioxidant capacity. Oxidative stress damages the sperm membrane and DNA, and reduces sperm viability and motility. Hence, the fertilizing capacity of semen is reduced and the risk of inadequate implantation or defective embryo development after ICSI may be increased.

Management of the male partner must address these aspects. Aside from treatment and recommendations regarding causal and coincidental factors, it may be considered advisable to administer nutritional supplements rich in antioxidants (Christophe et al., 1998; Zalata et al., 1998; Geva et al., 1996; Vezina et al., 1996; Kessopoulou et al., 1995; Fraga et al., 1991; 1996) and particular essential fatty acids (Christophe et al., 1998; Zalata et al., 1998).

The flowcharts (Figs. 4.1 and 4.2) suggest a strategy for management, based on current best evidence and cost-

41

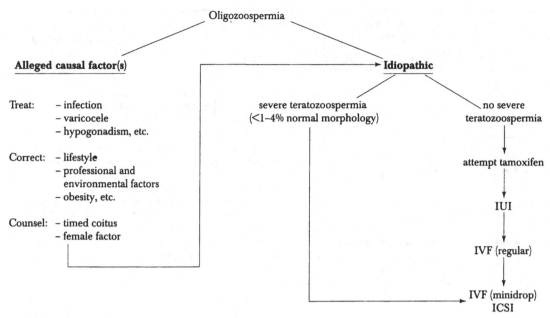

Fig. 4.2. Management of oligozoospermia.

effectiveness calculations. The proposed treatment strategy should be considered as a general guideline, and its application should be adapted depending on local circumstances (availability of microsurgery, IVF/ICSI facilities, etc.), and on the specific characteristics of the couple (previous treatments, age of both partners, duration of infertility, female pathology, etc.).

An independent effect of IUI, IVF and ovulation induction on neonatal morbidity cannot be ruled out, but most of the impact appears to be mediated by multiplicity and immaturity. Reducing the number of medically induced multiple pregnancies is the most effective prevention of neonatal morbidity related to these treatments (Addor et al., 1998).

Certain treatments must be considered experimental, in spite of their widespread application, since their long-term outcome regarding health and reproductive function of the offspring is not known. Careful follow-up of pregnancies and the offspring is mandatory.

Given the high success rates now being achieved using ICSI, there is an increasingly common trend for ICSI to be used as the treatment of choice. More disturbingly, there is a trend for infertile couples to be referred directly for ICSI treatment after an initial infertility consultation, in the belief that this is the most cost-effective approach to achieving the desired endpoint of a pregnancy. However, ICSI treatment is the most labour-intensive, invasive and expensive form of assisted conception treatment and is unwarranted for many couples (Mortimer, 1999). Several studies have suggested that ICSI is less cost-effective than varicocele treatment, vasectomy reversal, tamoxifen therapy and IUI (Schlegel, 1997; Pavlovich & Schlegel, 1997; Comhaire et al., 1996).

Although initial reports on birth defects in children born after ICSI have been reassuring, the results of a recent reanalysis of data indicate that ICSI may be associated with an increased incidence of both major and minor congenital anomalies (Kurinczuk & Bower, 1997). ICSI also carries an increased risk of transmitting infertility to the male offspring through the transmission of chromosomal, genetic (Kent-First et al., 1996), and other abnormalities. A recent study found an increased incidence of chromosome abnormalities in both partners of couples undergoing ICSI treatment, and recommended that chromosome analysis should also be performed in the female partner of couples undergoing ICSI (van der Ven et al., 1998). Therefore, ICSI should only be used as a 'last resort' when less-invasive, lower cost treatments have failed, although it may be the only approach likely to achieve success in couples with extreme male factor infertility, even sterility (e.g. the use of epididymal or testicular spermatozoa in cases of azoospermia).

Based on case reports, spermatozoa with large heads, multiple tails or absent acrosomal cap should not be used for ICSI without adequate chromosomal investigation. Normally, spermatozoa with any morphological abnormalities should not be used for ICSI, but in some cases these are the only ones available.

Preimplantation diagnosis of embryos should be performed in all patients with genetic or chromosomal abnormality, X-linked or other serious diseases (for review see Lissens & Sermon, 1997).

4.2.1 Sexual and/or ejaculatory dysfunction

Sexual and/or ejaculatory dysfunction includes the following.

Sexual dysfunction

Physical and psychosexual causes for inadequate erection and/or inadequate frequency of sexual intercourse.

(*a*) Inadequate coital erection
Management
- Assess organic and/or psychological causes.
- Treat underlying systemic, iatrogenic, urological, vascular, metabolic, neurological or endocrine causes.
- Attempt treatment with gonadotrophins if testosterone is low and LH is not elevated (hypogonadotrophic hypogonadism). Androgen replacement therapy can be considered if testosterone is low and LH is elevated, or if treatment with gonadotrophins remains ineffective. However, since high dose androgen treatment may suppress spermatogenesis, it should be considered with due care in case fertility is required.
- Associate counselling and psychotherapy.
- Consider intracavernosal injection with either papaverin, prostaglandin E_1, or pure alphalytic drugs, or medical treatment with an oral phosphodiesterase inhibitor.

(*b*) Inadequate frequency or incorrect timing of intercourse.
Management
- Treat by counselling.

NB Timing of intercourse should be around the day of ovulation. Ovulation may be detected by a change in basal body temperature (a chart may be used, but this rather unreliable), changes in cervical mucus, hormonal changes, or by suitable kits.

Ejaculatory disturbance
Coitus takes place normally but either no ejaculation takes place (anejaculation) or ejaculation occurs outside of the vagina due to either functional or anatomical reasons, e.g. hypospadias;

(*a*) Anejaculation
Management
- Assess organic or psychological causes.
- Treat underlying pathology.
- Intrauterine insemination or, in cases of failed IUI or poor semen quality, IVF or ICSI using the partner's semen obtained after vibro-massage or electro-ejaculation. If these methods fail, assisted reproduction using spermatozoa from the epididymis, the vas deferens or the testis (but this may induce iatrogenic obstruction).

(*b*)   Retrograde ejaculation

A specific form of ejaculatory disturbance where the semen is not ejaculated outside of the body but into the urinary bladder. In such cases the patient presents with aspermia or, when partial, small ejaculate volume with severe oligozoospermia. The postorgasm urine contains many spermatozoa.

Management

- Treat the causal factor whenever possible. In some cases with retrograde ejaculation as a result of resection of the paraaortic lymph nodes and damage to the systemic nervous system, α-mimetic drugs may restore antegrade ejaculation (Kohn & Schill, 1994).
- Artificial insemination (IUI) or assisted reproduction using spermatozoa recovered from alkalinized postorgasm urine or from the vas deferens, the epididymis or the testis if required.

NB Systemic alkalinization of urine may achieved by drinking a solution containing 3 to 5 g of sodium bicarbonate in 250 ml water on the morning of recovery of spermatozoa from urine. Alternatively, the patient is instructed to take 2 tablespoonfuls of sodium bicarbonate in a glass of water every 2 hours beginning 8 to 12 h before the recovery of spermatozoa from urine is required. If the urine sample pH is between 7.6 and 8.1 and the osmolarity is 300 to 500 mOsm/l, then the patient is asked to masturbate and then urinate in two separate vials containing buffered medium. The osmolarity of urine can be decreased by drinking increased amounts of water (for further details see Urry et al., 1986; Yavetz et al., 1994). Spermatozoa may also be recovered from the urinary bladder by catheterization and washing the bladder with appropriate medium. Sperm preparation and insemination must be performed as soon as possible.

All the following diagnoses require the presence of adequate sexual and ejaculatory function.

4.2.2   Immunological cause

This is diagnosed when 50% or more of motile spermatozoa are found to be coated with antibodies in at least one semen sample. The diagnosis should be confirmed by additional tests which assess the biological importance of antibodies (see Management).

Management

- Assess biological importance of antibodies by sperm–cervical mucus contact tests, either the postcoital test (PCT) in vivo or the sperm–cervical mucus contact (SCMC) test in vitro (see *WHO Laboratory Manual for the Examination of Human Semen and Sperm–Cervical Mucus Interaction* (CUP, 4th edn, 1999).
- Treat contributory conditions such as varicocele, infection or partial obstruction if spermatozoa are abnormal.
- Perform intrauterine insemination (IUI) of spermatozoa collected in culture medium ideally containing 0.3% (w/v) albumin and selected using one of the techniques described in Appendix IV.
- If IUI is unsuccessful after six cycles, or if sperm quality is severely deficient (see Figs. 4.1 and 4.2), perform IVF or ICSI as indicated.

NB There are few published large series of cases with an immunological cause (Mahmoud et al., 1996; Vazquez-Levin et al., 1997; Ombelet et al., 1997; Pagidas et al., 1994; Lahteenmaki, 1993). In general, IUI appears to be more successful when sperm characteristics are higher than the reference values (Appendix III) and when antisperm antibodies are directed against midpiece or tail. If antisperm antibodies are directed against the head or the entire spermatozoon, IUI may be less successful, although it can still be attempted if less than approximately 80% of the spermatozoa react in the MAR or Immunobead test. The probability of success by IUI is so low as to render this treatment unwarranted in cases with immunological cause and sperm characteristics well below the reference values, or sperm antibodies directed against the head or entire spermatozoon in more than approximately 80% of cells. In these cases IVF, possibly using increased sperm numbers, or ICSI should be more appropriate (Mortimer, 1999).

4.2.3 No demonstrable cause

This diagnosis is valid only if sexual and ejaculatory function are adequate and the semen classification is normal.

Management

- Assess female causes.
- If no female cause is detected, then treat long-standing unexplained infertility by assisted reproduction.

- Some authors recommend that the postcoital test (PCT) should be performed but the interpretation of its result is uncertain (*WHO Laboratory Manual for the Examination of Human Semen and Sperm–Cervical Mucus Interaction* (CUP, 4th edn, 1999).

4.2.4 Isolated seminal plasma abnormalities

These include normal spermatozoa but abnormalities in the physical, biochemical or bacteriological composition of the seminal plasma, or increased number of white blood cells or agglutination with a negative Immunobead or mixed antiglobulin reaction (MAR) test in patients with normal spermatozoa. These patients do not fulfil the criteria for the diagnosis of male accessory gland infection or any other pathology. The significance as a cause of infertility of isolated abnormalities in the seminal plasma is not known.

Management

- Assess female cause.
- Consider intracervical or intrauterine insemination of selected spermatozoa (in case of high ejaculate volume the sperm-rich first portion of the split ejaculate may be used), or assisted reproduction.

All the following aetiological diagnoses are only made if sexual and ejaculatory function are adequate and the semen classification is azoospermia or abnormal spermatozoa.

4.2.5 Iatrogenic causes

These are coded when the abnormal spermatozoa are considered to be due to medical or surgical causes.

This diagnosis requires the following to be true:

- history of medical treatment with possible adverse effect on fertility;
- and/or history of surgery with possible adverse effect on fertility.

Management

- Replace toxic medication by alternative treatment whenever possible.
- Perform sperm banking before chemotherapy or radiotherapy.

- Microscopically reverse vasectomy.

  If vasectomy reversal fails, treat as idiopathic azoospermia or oligozoospermia but genetic evaluation may be omitted (see Figs. 4.1 and 4.2)

NB Some authors suggest a second trial of microscopic vasectomy reversal may be worthwhile since they found it to be more cost effective than ICSI with epididymal spermatozoa (Donovan et al., 1998).

- Treat as an idiopathic abnormality according to semen quality (see below: idiopathic oligo-, astheno-, terato- and azoospermia).

4.2.6 Systemic causes

These should be recorded either if abnormal spermatozoa are considered to be related to a systemic disease and/or excessive alcohol consumption and/or drug abuse and/or environmental factors and/or recent high fever, or if the patient has immotile cilia syndrome (asthenozoospermia with less than 10% progressive motility and a history of chronic upper respiratory tract disease).

This diagnosis requires the following to be true:

- history of systemic disease;
- and/or high fever in the last 6 months;
- and/or environmental and/or occupational factors;
- and/or excessive consumption of alcohol and/or other life style factor(s) (e.g. smoking);
- and/or drug abuse.

Management

- Treat underlying disorder, avoid deleterious environmental influences, prohibit alcohol or drug abuse, and correct other life style factor(s).
- Treat as idiopathic oligozoospermia.
- Immotile cilia syndrome: The diagnosis is preferably confirmed by electron microscopy. Consider ICSI only after thorough counselling.

4.2.7 Congenital abnormalities

These include a history or clinical evidence of testicular maldescent, karyotype abnormalities, azoospermia due to congenital agenesis of the seminal vesicles and/or vasa deferentia and other congenital diseases.

Testicular maldescent

This diagnosis requires the following to be true:

- history of testicular maldescent;
- and/or abnormal testicular site and both testes palpable;
- and/or no history of testicular damage and at least one testis non-palpable;
- no history of surgery – orchiectomy.

Management

Correct testicular maldescent surgically if present after puberty in men up to 32 years of age; a patient with undescended testis after the age of 32 years is at greater risk of death from surgery than from testicular malignancy (Farrer et al., 1985). Perform testicular biopsy once (at least in cases with azoospermia or severe oligozoospermia) to exclude carcinoma in situ.

- Treat concomitant pathology such as varicocele or infection.
- Treat as an idiopathic abnormality according to semen quality (see below: idiopathic oligo-, astheno-, terato- and azoospermia).

Karyotype abnormalities

This diagnosis requires the following to be true:

- abnormal leukocyte karyotype;
- and/or Y chromosome microdeletions.

Management

- Propose artificial insemination using donor semen or adoption if karyotype abnormalities.
- In case of Klinefelter syndrome and its mosaic variants, and in cases of Y-chromosome gene deletion, ICSI with ejaculated or testicular spermatozoa can be considered. Since, however, there is a serious risk of transmitting the genetic defect, and therefore to transferring infertility to (male) offspring, the couple must receive thorough counselling beforehand (see General comments, p. 58).

Azoospermia due to congenital bilateral agenesis of the vasa deferentia

This diagnosis requires the following to be true:

- ejaculate volume <2 ml
  and pH <7;
- or vasa deferentia non-palpable (both sides).
  Management
  - In the case of congenital agenesis of the vasa deferentia, perform genetic analysis of both partners (for cystic fibrosis in particular) and consider ICSI with testicular or epididymal spermatozoa after genetic counselling. Preimplantation diagnosis may be mandatory if genetic defects are found in both partners.

Other congenital diseases

- Neurological and metabolic disorders. The description and diagnosis of these diseases is outside the scope of this work. Management should depend on the risk and mode of transmission to the offspring, the availability of preimplantation and prenatal diagnosis and semen quality (Hausmanowa-Petrusewicz et al., 1983; Malandrini et al., 1993; Brennemann et al., 1997; Futterweit & Mechanick, 1987).
- Immotile cilia syndrome (see Systemic causes p. 48);
- Kallmann syndrome (see Endocrine causes p. 54).

4.2.8 Acquired testicular damage

This should be recorded when the abnormal spermatozoa are considered to be due to either parotitis with orchitis, or pathology possibly causing testicular damage resulting in either a testicular volume of less than 15 ml or one or both testes being non-palpable.

This diagnosis requires the following to be true:

- history of pathology possibly causing testicular damage;
- and at least one testis with a volume of <15 ml or non-palpable.
  Management
  - Treat as an idiopathic abnormality according to semen quality (see below: idiopathic oligo-, astheno-, terato- and a-zoospermia).

4.2.9 Varicocele

Varicocele (either palpable or subclinical) must be associated with abnormal semen analysis to be accepted as a cause of infertility. If a man with varicocele has normal semen analysis, the varicocele is not considered to be the cause of infertility and the patient is coded as having no demonstrable abnormalities.

The role of varicocele in the aetiology of male infertility is controversial but analysis of the WHO data clearly shows that presence of varicocele relates to semen abnormalities, decreased testicular volume, and decline of Leydig cell function. (WHO, 1992a). Several reports suggest that men with varicocele also have an increased incidence of coincidental accessory gland infection (WHO, 1987), epididymal pathology (Gerris et al., 1988) or immunological factor (WHO, 1987; Gilbert et al., 1989; Golomb et al., 1986). Varicocele may be associated with a premature decrease in serum testosterone levels and with sexual dysfunction later in life (Comhaire & Vermeulen, 1975).

Several controlled studies have been performed, aiming at the assessment of a possible effect of varicocele treatment. Two of these are single centre studies and include a sufficient number of cases for valid statistical analysis. In the first study, surgically treated varicocele cases had a low pregnancy rate (10%) similar to that of untreated controls (Nilsson et al., 1979). In the second study, a prospective randomized trial, surgical treatment was equivalent to couple counselling, resulting in approximately 30% pregnancies after one year in both groups (Nieschlag et al., 1995).

WHO has organized a multicentre, prospective, randomized trial including infertile couples where the male partner had moderate oligozoospermia (5 to 20×10^6/ml) and a grade II or III varicocele. Immediate treatment was significantly more effective than delaying treatment for 1 year in attaining pregnancy, as well as in terms of pregnancy rate per cycle (fecundability), time to pregnancy and overall pregnancy rate (Hargreave, 1996).

Several studies have compared the outcome of surgical or radiological treatment of large versus small or subclinical varicoceles, and found no differences in results among cases with total testicular volume was within the normal range (30 ml or more) (Nieschlag et al., 1993; McClure et al., 1991; Comhaire & Kunnen, 1985). Therefore, varicocele treatment is considered acceptable in cases with no other cause of infertility in both partners, and moderate oligozoospermia, normal testicular volume and a varicocele.

Management

- Confirm the diagnosis of subclinical and grade I varicocele by additional investigations (see p. 31).
- Treat varicocele by transcatheter embolization or surgery.
- If no pregnancy occurs after 12 to 24 months following a successful varicocele repair, treat as an idiopathic abnormality according to semen quality (see idiopathic oligozoospermia p. 55).

NB Treatment of varicocele is of little benefit in terms of occurrence of subsequent pregnancy if there is one of the following combinations:

- grade I or subclinical varicoceles and (severely) reduced total testicular volume (<30 ml)
- azoospermia and normal testicular volume and normal FSH (suspect obstruction)
- azoospermia and elevated FSH, indicating severe damage of the seminiferous epithelium.

4.2.10 Male accessory gland infection (MAGI)

Sexually transmitted diseases and male accessory gland infection may impair male fertility through the following mechanisms:

- by increasing the production of reactive oxygen species by polymorphonuclear leukocytes in semen;
- by causing inflammatory lesions of the epididymis resulting in obstructive azoospermia or epididymal dysfunction;
- by stimulating antisperm antibody production;
- by causing urethritis, urethral strictures and ejaculatory disturbance.

Excess numbers of white blood cells may by themselves exert an unfavourable effect on the viability, motility, fertilizing capacity and the DNA composition of spermatozoa because of reactive oxygen species (Aitken & Clarkson, 1987; Zalata et al., 1995).

The diagnosis is given if the patient has oligo- or astheno- or teratozoospermia and fulfils the following criteria (Comhaire et al., 1980; Fari et al., 1976):

Group A. History/physical signs
- History of: urinary infection, epididymitis, sexually transmitted disease;
- Physical signs: thickened or tender epididymis, thickened vas deferens, abnormal rectal examination.

Group B. Urine after prostatic massage
- Abnormal urine after prostatic massage;
- Positive culture for *Chlamydia trachomatis,* or *Chlamydia trachomatis* DNA detected by PCR, LCR, or antigen detection by immunofluorescence or ELISA.

Group C. Ejaculate signs
- Elevated number of peroxidase positive white blood cells;
- Culture with significant growth of pathogenic bacteria;
- Positive culture for *Chlamydia trachomatis,* or *Chlamydia trachomatis* DNA detected by PCR, LCR, or antigen detection by immunofluorescence or ELISA;
- Abnormal appearance and/or viscosity and/or pH and/or abnormal biochemistry of the seminal plasma and/or high levels of inflammatory markers or highly elevated reactive oxygen species.

The diagnosis requires at least two signs:
- two signs each from a different group, e.g. thickened vas deferens with abnormal biochemistry of seminal plasma (or any other combination);
- or at least two ejaculate signs in each ejaculate.

Management
- If *Escherichia coli, Proteus* or *Klebsiella* spp.: treat with a fluorinated quinolone for 20 days.
- If *Streptococcus* spp.: administer aminopenicillin or doxycycline for 20 days.
- If *Chlamydia trachomatis*: treat with a fluorinated quinolone for 20 days (female partner should be treated concomitantly).
- If sperm quality remains abnormal, treat as an idiopathic abnormality according to semen quality (see below: idiopathic oligo-, astheno-, terato- and a-zoospermia).

NB Patients fulfilling the criteria of MAGI, including abnormal semen analysis, will only occasionally have their semen quality restored to normal after antibiotic treatment. Treatment aims at the elimination of bacterial infestation and reduction of the number of white blood cells, which may then improve the fertilizing capacity of spermatozoa during treatment by means of IUI or IVF. Several studies suggest that treatment with antioxidants may further reduce damage caused by reactive oxygen species to the sperm membrane and DNA, but the possible effect of this on fertility requires further investigation.

4.2.11 Endocrine causes

Patients with endocrine causes of infertility may present with signs of hypogonadism, but the diagnosis is made in cases with a normal or low serum FSH and low plasma testosterone or repeatedly elevated prolactin values. Further investigations should be performed to detect the precise cause. These patients may sometimes present with sexual or ejaculatory dysfunction. In this case they must be categorized accordingly.

This diagnosis requires the following to be true:

- low plasma testosterone with serum FSH not elevated;
- and/or elevated repeat prolactin.

Management

- Assess causal factor.
- Treat hypogonadotrophic hypogonadism with gonadotrophins.
- Assess and treat cause of hyperprolactinaemia, administer dopominergic medication when indicated, e.g. bromocriptine or cabergoline.
- Give complementary gonadotrophin treatment if required.
- Offer assisted reproduction if persistent oligozoospermia or azoospermia.
- If repeated failure of fertilization, offer artificial insemination of donor semen or adoption.

Descriptive diagnoses may only be given if none of the preceding diagnoses is applicable and the semen classification is oligo-, astheno-, terato- or a-zoospermia. Sexual and ejaculatory function must be adequate.

4.2.12   Idiopathic oligozoospermia

This is accepted if sperm concentration is less than 20×10^6/ml but more than 0.0×10^6/ml and none of the other diagnoses is applicable.

Management

- Treat with anti-oestrogen if serum FSH is not elevated.

  When tamoxifen is given in a dose of 20 mg per day, no oestrogenic effect can be detected in men (Comhaire, 1976). This treatment was found to increase sperm concentration significantly in two double-blind, placebo-controlled studies (Adamopoulos et al., 1997; Kotoulas et al., 1994). Also, three double-blind studies indicated the probability of conception to be increased (RR = 2.07), although statistical significance was not reached in meta-analysis (95% CI = 0.84–5.11) (O'Donovan et al., 1993; AinMelk et al., 1987; Torök, 1985; Krause et al., 1992).

  Therefore, while treatment with tamoxifen may be considered appropriate in cases with idiopathic oligozoospermia, particularly when sperm motility and morphology are not severely deficient, further studies are needed.

- Consider intrauterine insemination or assisted reproduction depending on semen characteristics (see General comments p. 58 and Figs. 4.1 and 4.2, and Appendix IV).

  NB Treatment with clomiphene citrate, which is a racemic mixture of Em-isomer that displays 'pure' anti-oestrogen effects with the Zu-isomer that has rather pronounced intrinsic oestrogenic effects, was found to be ineffective (World Health Organization, 1992b). Also, literature meta-analysis of placebo-controlled studies in men with oligo-astheno-terato-zoospermia (Gerris, 1997; AinMelk et al., 1987; Torök, 1985; Krause et al., 1992), indicate that clomiphene therapy does not increase pregnancy rate.

4.2.13   Idiopathic asthenozoospermia

This requires a normal sperm concentration, but a low proportion of spermatozoa with progressive motility in relation to the reference values of the laboratory, and none of the other diagnoses is applicable.

Management

- Evaluate repeat semen analysis after short interval (e.g. on the same or next day).
- Offer intrauterine insemination of selected spermatozoa or assisted reproduction depending on sperm characteristics after sperm selection procedures (see Fig. 4.1).
- If repeated failure of fertilization, offer artificial insemination of donor semen or adoption.

4.2.14 Idiopathic teratozoospermia

This requires normal concentration and motility but low morphology (proportion of spermatozoa with normal morphology below the reference values of the laboratory), and none of the other diagnoses is applicable.

Management

This is dependent on the severity of teratozoospermia.

- If moderate teratozoospermia, attempt IUI or IVF.
- In cases with severe teratozoospermia or failed IUI or IVF, attempt IVF with ICSI (see General comments, p. 58).
- If repeated failure of fertilization, offer artificial insemination of donor semen or adoption.

4.2.15 Idiopathic cryptozoospermia

This is diagnosed if no spermatozoa are seen in the fresh sample, but a few spermatozoa are recovered in the sediment after centrifugation, and none of the other diagnoses is applicable.

Management

- ICSI using spermatozoa found in semen after thorough genetic evaluation and counselling (see General comments, p. 58).

4.2.16 Obstructive azoospermia

This is diagnosed if the semen classification is azoospermia and the testicular biopsy reveals a full spermatogenic complement in any of the seminiferous tubules (see Testicular biopsy, p. 33).

This diagnosis requires the following to be true:

- spermatozoa present in the testicular biopsy;
- and total testicular volume >30 ml or single testis volume >15 ml;

- and normal plasma FSH;
- and none of the other diagnoses applicable.

  Management
  - Perform surgical scrotal exploration and attempt microsurgical repair.
  - Consider IVF, preferably ICSI, using epididymal or testicular spermatozoa after thorough genetic evaluation and counselling.
  - Offer artificial insemination using donor semen, or adoption.

4.2.17 Idiopathic azoospermia

This is diagnosed when the patient's azoospermia is of unknown origin, i.e. patients with low or normal testicular volume or elevated FSH and spermatozoa are absent in any of the seminiferous tubules.

This diagnosis requires the following to be true:

- elevated serum FSH;
- and/or total testicular volume ≤30 ml or single testis volume ≤15 ml;
- and spermatozoa absent in the testicular biopsy;
- and none of the other diagnoses applicable.

Management

There is no treatment for idiopathic and complete spermatogenic and maturation arrest or Sertoli-cell only syndrome (germ cell aplasia). In cases presenting with focal spermatogenesis or isolated tubules with full spermatogenesis, ICSI with testicular spermatozoa can be offered after thorough genetic evaluation and counselling. However, these cases do not fulfil the criteria for idiopathic azoospermia. Treatment by intracytoplasmic injection of spermatids or spermatid nuclei should be considered experimental.

- Offer artificial insemination using donor spermatozoa, or adoption.

NB Polyzoospermia

The significance of polyzoospermia as a cause of infertility is debatable (Glezerman et al., 1982; Testart et al., 1983). The reported incidence of polyzoospermia in subfertile men varies from 0.2% to 13% (Amelar et al., 1979; Merino & Carranza-Lira, 1995; Tournaye et al., 1997b).

Polyzoospermia has been repeatedly associated with reduced spontaneous fertility and increased rates of spontaneous abortion (Homonnai et al; 1980; Glezerman et al., 1982).

Studies indicate defective sperm capacitation (Kholkute et al., 1992) and acrosome reaction (Schill & Feifel, 1984; Topfer-Petersen et al., 1987; Schill et al., 1988; Kholkute et al., 1992), and decreased concentration of sperm acrosin in men with polyzoospermia (Calamera et al., 1987). Polyzoospermic men did not appear to have defective spermatozoal fertilizing capacity, as assessed by the heterologous sperm–ova penetration bioassay (Chan et al., 1986). Other reported abnormalities in polyzoospermic men include low levels of sperm adenosine triphosphate (Calamera et al., 1987) and DNA (for review see in Tournaye et al., 1997b) and prostaglandin E (Bendvold et al., 1987).

Studies on the outcome of conventional IVF in cases with polyzoospermia show neither a reduction in spermatozoal fertilizing capacity (Testart et al., 1983; Tournaye et al., 1997b), nor an increase in pregnancy wastage in cycles in which a pregnancy was obtained (Tournaye et al., 1997b).

Methods reported for the management of infertility associated with polyzoospermia include precoital dilutional douching, in vitro seminal fluid dilution and artificial insemination (Amelar et al; 1979), and conventional IVF (Tournaye et al., 1997b).

4.3   GENERAL COMMENTS

4.3.1   General treatment strategy

Management of male infertility aims at treating the male patient in an attempt to improve his semen quality and/or at making optimal use of his spermatozoa. Treatment of a causal factor or of idiopathic oligozoospermia may result in such improvement that the probability of natural conception is increased. It may also increase the probability of success of certain techniques of assisted reproduction and 'downgrade' the method needed to achieve pregnancy from the more sophisticated, costly and invasive mode (ICSI, TESE. . .) to less invasive techniques (IUI or conventional IVF). In doing so, treatment of the male may reduce the risk of treatment for the female partner and the offspring, decrease the cost of treatment for the couple and for society, and, sometimes, increase the effective cumulative pregnancy since, for example, IUI can easily be repeated in subsequent cycles, whereas IVF (and ICSI) is usually performed at intervals of several months and drop-out rates are high (Comhaire et al., 1995; Land et al., 1997).

4.3.2 Notes on assisted reproduction

Intrauterine insemination of selected spermatozoa (see Appendix IV) is successful, provided a minimum number of progressively motile spermatozoa are available in the native ejaculate and/or after sperm selection (Byrd et al., 1987; Horvath et al., 1989; Brasch et al., 1994; Aribarg & Sukcharoen, 1995; Berg et al., 1997; for reviews see Schoysman and Daniore, 1991; Cohlen et al., 1995; Ford et al., 1997; Keck et al., 1997).

Depending on the technique of morphology assessment, there is a lower limit for the proportion of spermatozoa with normal morphology below which neither IUI nor conventional IVF will be successful. This limit is usually set at between 1 and 4% normal forms, but depends on the criteria used for sperm morphology evaluation (Ombelet et al., 1997a).

Conventional IVF generates a poor success rate in cases with extreme teratozoospermia, and in patients where sperm deficiency results from testicular maldescent or other congenital abnormalities. Poor results of conventional IVF have also been associated with acrosome abnormalities.

ICSI can be applied successfully in cases with severe sperm deficiency resulting from acquired pathology. ICSI treatment in cases with congenital abnormalities or idiopathic sperm deficiency or azoospermia includes an inherent risk of transmission of genetic defects. ICSI treatment in such cases is admissible only after thorough genetic investigation (including searching for Y chromosome microdeletions and possibly cystic fibrosis gene mutations) and genetic counselling. Further research is needed to evaluate the possible risks of spermatid injection, which should currently be considered as experimental.

For the management of a patient with azoospermia, see also Fig. 4.1. The assessment of α-glucosidase activity in seminal plasma of azoospermic men, together with measurement of testicular volume (and by inference epididymal size), serum FSH and testosterone, can help in differentiating between the major causes of this condition. Bilateral obstruction between the cauda epididymidis and the ejaculatory duct is associated with low levels of seminal α-glucosidase (Guérin et al., 1986; Cooper et al., 1988; 1990; Mahmoud et al., 1998a). The operative setting may be planned according to the likely diagnosis and intended intervention, e.g. facilities for scrotal exploration and microsurgical reconstruction when an obstruction is suspected.

Appendix I
Data collection form and flowchart

Male partner

	Day	Month	Year
Date of history taking			

	Day	Month	Year
Date of birth			

FERTILITY HISTORY

Infertility   □ primary
                           □ secondary

Duration of infertility   ☐☐☐ months

Months since last
impregnation   ☐☐☐

Previous investigation(s) and/or
treatments for infertility   □ no   □ yes*

* Please provide additional information.

PATHOLOGY OR TREATMENT(S) WITH POSSIBLE INFLUENCE ON FERTILITY

History of medical disease	☐ no	☐ diabetes	☐ tuberculosis
		☐ chronic respiratory tract disease	☐ fibrocystic disease of the pancreas
		☐ neurologic disease	☐ other*
History of medical treatment	☐ no	☐ yes*	
High fever in past 6 months	☐ no	☐ yes*	
History of surgery	☐ no	☐ urethral strictures	☐ hypospadias
		☐ prostatectomy	☐ bladder neck operation
		☐ vasectomy	
		☐ inguinal hernia	☐ hydrocelectomy
		☐ sympathectomy	☐ other*
History of urinary infection	☐ no	☐ yes*	
History of sexually transmitted disease	☐ no	☐ syphilis	☐ gonorrhoea
		☐ chlamydia	☐ other*

side: left – right

			left	right
History of epididymitis	☐ no	☐ yes*	☐	☐
History of pathology possibly causing testicular damage	☐ no	☐ orchitis: mumps	☐	☐
		☐ orchitis: other*	☐	☐
		☐ injury*	☐	☐
		☐ torsion*	☐	☐
History of varicocele treatment	☐ no	☐ yes*	☐	☐
History of testicular maldescent	☐ no	☐ yes	☐	☐
Treatment for testicular maldescent		☐ none	☐ medical	☐ surgical
		☐☐ Age at treatment		

OTHER FACTORS WITH POSSIBLE INFLUENCE ON FERTILITY

Environmental and/or occupational factors	☐ no	☐ heat	☐ other*
		☐ toxic factors	
Excess consumption of alcohol	☐ no	☐ yes*	
Drug abuse	☐ no	☐ yes*	
Tobacco smoking	☐ no	☐ yes	number of cigarettes/day ☐☐
			number of years smoking ☐☐

SEXUAL AND EJACULATORY FUNCTION

Average frequency of intercourse per month	☐ normal	☐ inadequate
Erection	☐ normal	☐ inadequate*
Ejaculation	☐ normal	☐ inadequate*

* Please provide additional information.

GENERAL PHYSICAL EXAMINATION

Height (cm) ☐☐☐

Weight (kg) ☐☐☐

Blood pressure (mm HG) ☐☐☐ ☐☐☐

General physical examination ☐ normal ☐ abnormal*

Signs of virilisation ☐ normal ☐ hypoandrogenism*

Gynaecomastia ☐ absent

☐ Tanner stage

URO-GENITAL EXAMINATION

Penis ☐ normal ☐ scars ☐ hypospadias
                     ☐ plaques ☐ other*

side: left – right

Testes ☐ both palpable non-palpable ☐ ☐

Site ☐ both normal abnormal* ☐ ☐

Volume (ml) ☐☐ left ☐☐ right

Epididymides ☐ both normal thickened ☐ ☐
                             tender ☐ ☐
                             cystic ☐ ☐
                             non-palpable ☐ ☐

Vasa deferentia ☐ both normal thickened ☐ ☐
                               non-palpable ☐ ☐

Scrotal swelling ☐ none hydrocele ☐ ☐
                        hernia ☐ ☐

Varicocele ☐ none grade III ☐ ☐
                  grade II ☐ ☐
                  grade I ☐ ☐
                  subclinical ☐ ☐

Inguinal examination ☐ normal lymphadenopathy ☐ ☐
                            infectious scars ☐ ☐
                            surgical scars ☐ ☐
                            hernia ☐ ☐

Rectal examination ☐ normal

– prostate ☐ soft swelling ☐ tender
           ☐ hard swelling ☐ other

– seminal vesicles ☐ palpable

Contact thermography ☐ normal ☐ abnormal*

ADDITIONAL INFORMATION

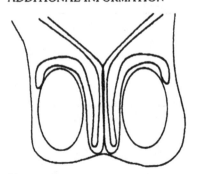

SEMEN ANALYSIS

	First analysis			Second analysis		
	Day	Month	Year	Day	Month	Year
Date						

Duration of abstinence (days)

Analysis of spermatozoa

Concentration ($\times 10^6$/ml)

Motility (%)
(a) rapid linear progression

(b) slow or non-linear progression   ☐ not done

(c) non-progressive motility

(d) immotile

Vitality (% live)   ☐ not done

Morphology (% normal forms)

Immunobead or MAR-test (% positive)

Agglutination   ☐ none   ☐ yes   ☐ none   ☐ yes

Seminal plasma analysis

Volume (ml)

Appearance and consistency   ☐ both normal   ☐ abnormal   ☐ both normal   ☐ abnormal

pH

Biochemistry   ☐ normal   ☐ abnormal   ☐ not done   ☐ normal   ☐ abnormal   ☐ not done

White blood cells ($\times 10^6$/ml)

Other round cells ($\times 10^6$/ml)

Culture   ☐ negative   ☐ positive   ☐ not done   ☐ negative   ☐ positive   ☐ not done

Semen centrifugation* spermatoza   ☐ present   ☐ absent   ☐ present   ☐ absent

• Only if no spermatozoa are detected during routine semen analysis.

SEMEN CLASSIFICATION

	First	Second
Antibody-coated spermatozoa	☐	☐
Normal semen	☐	☐
Normal spermatoza with agglutination, abnormal seminal plasma, or WBCs	☐	☐
Teratozoospermia	☐	☐
Asthenozoospermia	☐	☐
Oligozoospermia	☐	☐
Cryptozoospermia	☐	☐
Azoospermia	☐	☐
Aspermia	☐	☐

ADDITIONAL TESTS

	normal	abnormal*	not done
Prostatic expression fluid and/or urine after prostatic massage	☐ normal	☐ abnormal*	☐ not done
Post-orgasm urine	☐ no spermatozoa	☐ spermatozoa present	☐ not done
Screening blood and urine	☐ normal	☐ abnormal*	☐ not done
Plasma FSH (IU/l) ☐☐·☐	☐ normal	☐ abnormal*	☐ not done
Plasma testosterone (nmol/l) ☐☐☐·☐	☐ normal	☐ low	☐ not done
Prolactin (mU/l) ☐☐☐☐	☐ normal	☐ elevated	☐ not done
Repeat prolactin (mU/l) ☐☐☐☐	☐ normal	☐ elevated	☐ not done
Leucocyte karyotype	☐ normal	☐ abnormal*	☐ not done
Testicular biopsy	☐ spermatozoa present	☐ spermatozoa absent	☐ not done
Doppler echography	☐ normal	☐ abnormal*	☐ not done
Sella turcica	☐ normal	☐ enlarged	☐ not done
Additional investigations	☐ normal	☐ abnormal*	☐ not done

DIAGNOSIS

☐ Sexual and/or ejaculatory dysfunction
☐ Immunological causes
☐ No demonstrable cause
☐ Isolated seminal plasma abnormalities
☐ Iatrogenic causes
☐ Systemic causes
☐ Congenital abnormalities
☐ Acquired testicular damage

☐ Varicocele
☐ Male accessory gland infection
☐ Endocrine causes
☐ Idiopathic oligozoospermia
☐ Idiopathic asthenozoospermia
☐ Idiopathic teratozoospermia
☐ Idiopathic cryptozoospermia
☐ Obstructive azoospermia
☐ Idiopathic azoospermia

ADDITIONAL INFORMATION

DIAGNOSTIC FLOWCHART

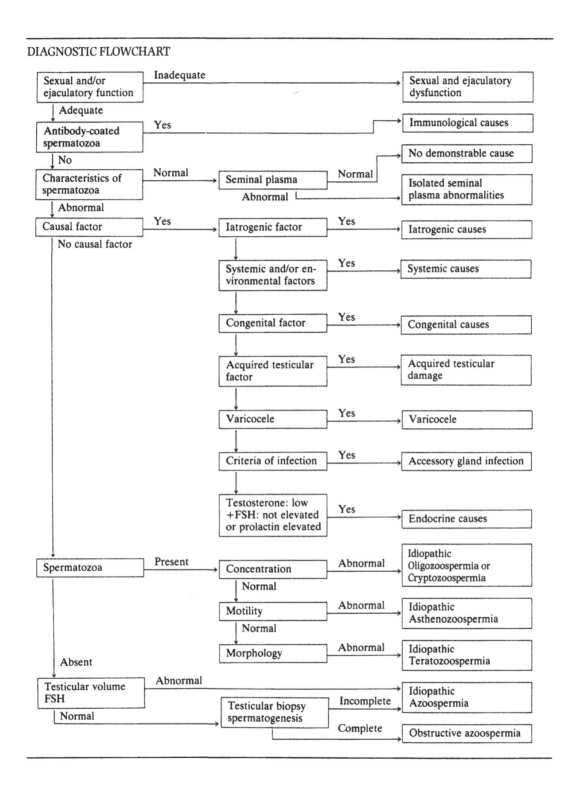

Appendix II
Tanner pubertal stage

Appendix II.1
Tanner pubertal stage

Fig. II.1.1. Standards of genital maturity in boys

Stage 1. Preadolescent. Testes, scrotum and penis are about same size and shape as in early childhood.

Stage 2. Scrotum and testes are slightly enlarged. The skin of the scrotum is reddened and changed in texture. There is little or no enlargement of the penis at this stage.

Stage 3. Penis is slightly enlarged, at first mainly in length. Testes and scrotum are further enlarged than in Stage 2.

Stage 4. Penis is further enlarged, with growth in breadth and development of glans. Testes and scrotum are further enlarged than in Stage 3: scrotal skin is darker than in earlier stages.

Stage 5. Genitalia are adult in size and shape.

Reproduced with permission from Tanner, J.M. (1962).

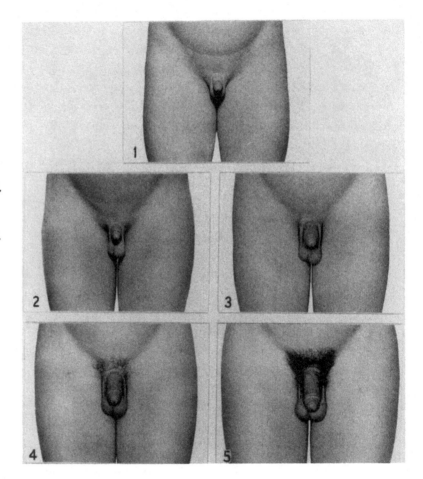

Fig. II.1.2. Standards for pubic hair ratings (*a*) in boys.

Stage 1. Preadolescent. The vellus over the pubes is not further developed than that over the abdominal wall, i.e. no pubic hair.

Stage 2. There is sparse growth of long, slightly pigmented downy hair, straight, or slightly curled, chiefly at the base of the penis.

Stage 3. The hair is considerably darker, coarser and more curled. It spreads sparsely over the junction of the pubes.

Stage 4. Hair is now adult in type, but the area covered is still considerably smaller than in the adult. There is no spread to the medial surface of the thighs.

Stage 5. The hair is adult in quantity and type with distribution of the horizontal (or classically 'feminine') pattern. Spread is to the medial surface of the thighs, but not up the linea alba or elsewhere above the base of the inverse triangle.

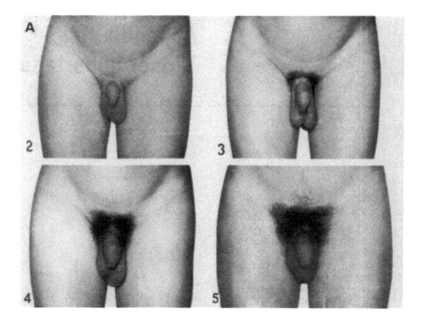

Appendix II.2
Tanner pubertal stage

Fig. II.2.1. Standards for breast development ratings (from Tanner, 1962).

Stage 1. Preadolescent. There is elevation of the papilla only.

Stage 3. Breast and areola are both enlarged and elevated more than in Stage 2, but with no separation of their contours.

Stage 4. The areola and papilla form a secondary mound projecting above the contour of the breast.

Stage 5. Mature stage. The papilla only projects, with the areola recessed to the general contour of the breast.

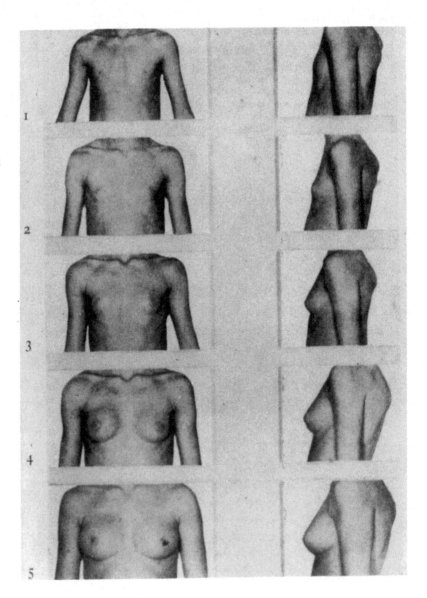

Appendix III
Reference values for semen variables

Each laboratory should determine its own reference ranges for each variable. For reference semen variables, specimens should be evaluated from men who have recently achieved a pregnancy, preferably within 12 months of the couple ceasing contraception, or prospective studies of fertility should be undertaken. The need for large numbers and the complex relationship between semen analysis results and fertilization, together with the time taken to achieve pregnancy, make these studies difficult to perform. Consequently, generally applicable reference ranges have not been established as they have for other laboratory tests. To date, no significant differences in semen variables have been found between races.

In this context the following reference ranges are given based on the clinical experience of many investigators from populations of healthy fertile men. Because these values are not the minimum semen values needed for conception, e.g. by evaluation of in vitro or in vivo fertility from a subfertile population, their categorization has been changed from 'normal' values to 'reference' values. Thus men with semen variables lower than those indicated in this manual may be fertile.

Reference values

Volume	2.0 ml or more
pH	7.2 or more
Sperm concentration	20×10^6 spermatozoa/ml or more
Total sperm number	40×10^6 spermatozoa per ejaculate or more
Motility	50% or more with progressive motility (grades 'a' and 'b') or 25% or more with rapid linear progression (grade 'a') within 60 minutes of ejaculation.
Morphology*	
Vitality	75% or more live, i.e. excluding dye
White blood cells	fewer than 1×10^6/ml
Immunobead test	fewer than 50% motile spermatozoa with beads bound
MAR test	fewer than 50% motile spermatozoa with adherent particles

*(a) Multicentre population-based studies using the methods of morphology assessment in the *WHO Laboratory Manual* (CUP, 4th edn, 1999), are now in progress.

(b) Data from assisted reproductive technology programmes suggest that, as sperm morphology falls below 15% normal forms using the methods and definitions described in the *WHO Laboratory Manual* (CUP, 4th edn, 1999), the fertilization rate in vitro decreases.

Appendix IV
Methods for spermatozoa selection for use in insemination or assisted reproduction

There are different methods for selecting spermatozoa for use in insemination or in assisted reproduction, including the direct swim-up from semen technique, glass wool and Sephadex filtration, and the use of density gradients. Percoll® is not available for the isolation of human spermatozoa for use in assisted reproductive technologies and it has been replaced by the use of silanized colloidal silica particles, for which there are several commercial sources. Swim-up and density gradients remove seminal plasma, whereas glass wool and Sephadex columns do not. The method of centrifugation–resuspension (simple sperm 'washing') is *not* recommended since it does not select spermatozoa of good quality, and results in oxidative stress that may affect IUI or IVF outcomes adversely. The term 'selected spermatozoa' used below refers to spermatozoa prepared by using the recommended techniques.

Treatment options should be based on results of a 'trial sperm preparation' to ascertain the treatment modalities that are feasible for the man (Mortimer, 1994). Cut-offs in terms of the numbers of progressively motile spermatozoa available from processing a man's ejaculate should be developed by each laboratory to guide patient management in terms of:

(a) the type(s) of assisted reproductive technology(ies) that can be used (e.g. IUI, GIFT, IVF or ICSI); and

(b) the type of IVF insemination that should be used (e.g. droplets under oil vs. open dishes or tubes).

Although sperm preparation often selects for morphologically normal spermatozoa, general experience has shown the most important sperm morphology information for patient management is that obtained from seminal populations, especially when the Teratozoospermia Index (TZI) is calculated. The actual number of motile spermatozoa to be used for IVF (or GIFT) may be increased to compensate for poorer sperm morphology; although this practice will be very dependent upon individual laboratories' experience. Some application of this process is shown in Figure 4.1.

Obviously, the final decisions in these matters must be taken in conjunction with considerations of female factors, such as tubal patency, ovulatory status, cycle regularity, age, etc. Also, antisperm antibodies in the female serum causing greater than 50% bead or particle binding, especially if head directed, contraindicate the use of female serum to supplement culture media for sperm preparation and IVF, whereas IUI and GIFT may be less successful.

With the publication of the 4th edition of its *Laboratory Manual for the Examination of Human Semen and Sperm–Cervical Mucus Interaction* (1999), the WHO has supported the use of Tygerberg Strict Criteria for the assessment of normal human sperm morphology. However, the Teratozoospermia Index (TZI) has been included to provide additional information to facilitate discrimination of the extent of impairment of sperm functional potential in men with very low numbers of normal spermatozoa. For example, the management of two men with, say, 4% normal forms may be differentiated using TZI values: if one has a TZI value of <1.7 he may be expected to achieve successful fertilization in vitro without recourse to ICSI (although IUI may be rather unsuccessful), but if the other has a TZI >1.9 he may well require ICSI in order to achieve fertilization of his partner's oocytes. Although each laboratory is recommended to establish its own criterion values to manage patients with teratozoospermia (*WHO Laboratory Manual for the Examination of Human Semen and Sperm–Cervical Mucus Interaction*, CUP, 4th edn, 1999), extreme teratozoospermia may be defined generally as 0% normal forms combined with TZI >1.7. Further studies and more extensive clinical experience will permit better definition of more widely applicable criterion values in the future as laboratories acquire greater experience in assessing sperm morphology to the new criteria, and as the impact of training courses, internal quality control and external quality assurance programmes become more widespread.

References

Abramsson L., Duchek M., Lundgren B. (1989). Conception rate for infertile couples. The importance of anamnesis and signs of genital disease in men with abnormal semen findings. *Scand. J. Urol. Nephrol.*, **23**: 165–171.

Adamopoulos D.A., Nicopoulou S., Kapolla N., Karamertzanis M., Andreou E. (1997). The combination of testosterone undecanoate with tamoxifen citrate enhances the effects of each agent given independently on seminal parameters in men with idiopathic oligozoospermia. *Fertil. Steril.*, **67**: 756–762.

Addor V., Santos-Eggimann B., Fawer C., Paccaud F., Calame A. (1998). Impact of infertility treatments on the health of newborns. *Fertil. Steril.*, **69**: 210–215.

Ain Melk Y., Belisle S., Carmel M., Jean-Pierre T. (1987). Tamoxifen citrate therapy in male infertility. *Fertil. Steril.*, **48**: 113–117.

Aitken R.J., Clarkson J.S. (1987). Cellular basis of defective sperm function and its association with the genesis of reactive oxygen species by human spermatozoa. *J. Reprod. Fertil.*, **81**: 459–469.

Amelar R.D., Dubin L., Quigley M.M., Schoenfeld C. (1979). Successful management of infertility due to polyzoospermia. *Fertil. Steril.*, **31**: 521–524.

Andreou E., Mahmoud A., Vermeulen L., Comhaire F. (1995). Comparison of different methods for the investigation of antisperm antibodies on spermatozoa, in seminal plasma and in serum. *Hum. Reprod.*, **10**: 125–131.

Aribarg A., Sukcharoen N. (1995). Intrauterine insemination of washed spermatozoa for treatment of oligozoospermia. *Int. J. Androl.*, **18** (Suppl. 1): 62–66.

Batata M.A., Whitmore W.F., Cun F.C. et al. (1980). Cryptorchidism and testicular cancer. *J. Urol.*, **124**: 382–387.

Bendvold E., Gottlieb C., Svanborg K., Bygdeman M., Eneroth P. (1987). Concentration of prostaglandins in seminal fluid of fertile men. *Int. J. Androl.*, **10**: 463–469.

Berg U., Brucker C., Berg F.D. (1997). Effect of motile sperm count after swim-up on outcome of intrauterine insemination. *Fertil. Steril.*, **67**: 747–750.

Bosl G.J., Motzer R.J. (1997). Testicular germ-cell cancer. *N. Eng. J. Med.*, **337** (4): 242–253.

Brasch J.G., Rawlins R., Tarchala S., Radwanska E. (1994). The relationship between total motile sperm count and success of intrauterine insemination. *Fertil. Steril.*, **62**: 150–154.

Brennemann W., Kohler W., Zierz S., Klingmuller D. (1997). Testicular dysfunction in adrenomyeloneuropathy. *Eur. J. Endocrinol.*, **137**: 34–39.

Byrd W., Ackerman G.E., Carr B.R., Edman C.D., Guzick D.S., McConnell J.D. (1987). Treatment of refractory infertility by transcervical intrauterine insemination of washed spermatozoa. *Fertil. Steril.*, **48**: 921–927.

Calamera J.C., Giovenco P., Brugo S., Dondero F., Nicholson R.F. (1987). Adenosine 5 triphosphate (ATP) content and acrosin activity in polyzoospermic subjects. *Andrologia*, **19**: 460–463.

Campbell H.E. (1959). The incidence of malignant growth of the undescended testicle: a reply and re-evaluation. *J. Urol.*, **81**: 563.

Chan S.Y., Tang L.C., Tang G.W., Ho P.C., Wang C. (1986). Spermatozoal fertilizing capacity in polyzoospermia: a preliminary study. *Andrologia*, **18**: 208–213.

Christophe A., Zalata A., Mahmoud A., Comhaire F. (1998). Fatty acid composition of sperm phospholipids and its nutritional implications. *Middle East Fertil. Soc. J.*, **3**: 46–53.

Close C.E., Roberts P.L., Berger R.E. (1990). Cigarettes, alcohol and marijuana are related to pyospermia in infertile men. *J. Urol.*, **144**: 900–903.

Cohlen B.J., te Velde E.R., van Kooij R.J. (1995). Is there still a place for intrauterine insemination as a treatment for male subfertility?. A review. *Int. J. Androl.*, **18** (Suppl. 2): 72–75.

Collins J.A., So Y., Wilson E.H., Wrixon W., Casper R.F. (1984). Clinical factors affecting pregnancy rates among infertile couples. *Can. Med. Assoc. J.*, **130**: 269–273.

Colpi G.M., Casella F., Zanollo A., Ballerini G., Balerna M., Campana A., Lange A (1987). Functional voiding disturbances of the ampullo-vesicular seminal tract: a cause of male infertility. *Acta Eur. Fertil.*, **18**: 165–179.

Comhaire F. (1976). Treatment of oligozoospermia with Tamoxifen. *Int. J. Fertil*, **21**: 232–238.

Comhaire F.H. (1996). Definition of infertility, subfertility and fecundability: methods to calculate the success rate of treatment. In *Male Infertility*. ed. F.H. Comhaire. Chapman & Hall, pp. 123–131.

Comhaire F. (1998). Pitfalls of evidence based medicine in andrology and assisted reproduction. *Studies in Profertility Series*, volume 8. *Modern ART in the 2000s. Andrology in the nineties* ed. W. Ombelet, E. Bosmans, H. Vandeput, A. Vereecken, M. Renier, E. Hoomans, The Parthenon Publishing Group, New York, London, pp. 45–52.

Comhaire F., Vermeulen A.(1975). Plasma testosterone in patients with varicocele and sexual inadequacy. *J. Clin. Endocrinol. Metab.*, **40**: 824–829.

Comhaire F.H., Kunnen M. (1985). Factors affecting the probability of conception after treatment of subfertile men with varicocele by transcatheter embolization with Bucrylate. *Fertil. Steril.*, **43**: 781–786.

Comhaire F., Verschraegen G., Vermeulen L. (1980). Diagnosis of accessory gland infection and its possible role in male infertility. *Int. J. Androl.*, **3**: 32–45.

Comhaire F.H., Vermeulen L., Schoonjans F. (1987). Reassessment of the accuracy of traditional sperm characteristics and adenosine triphosphate (ATP) in estimating the fertilizing potential of human semen in vivo. *Int. J. Androl,* **10**: 653–662.

Comhaire F., Milingos S., Liapi A., Gordts S., Campo R., Depypere H., Dhont M., Schoonjans F. (1995). The effective cumulative pregnancy rate of different modes of treatment of male infertility. *Andrologia,* **27**: 217–221.

Comhaire F., Zalata A., Mahmoud A. (1996). Critical evaluation of the effectiveness of different modes of treatment of male infertility. *Andrologia,* **28** (Suppl. 1): 31–35.

Cooper, T.G., Yeung, C.H., Nashan, D., Nieschlag, E. (1988). Epididymal markers in male infertility. *J. Androl.*, **9**: 91–101.

Cooper T.G., Yeung C.H., Nashan D., Jockenhovel F., Nieschlag E. (1990). Improvement in the assessment of human epididymal function by the use of inhibitors in the assay of alpha-glucosidase in seminal plasma. *Int. J. Androl.*, **13**: 297–305.

Cooper, T.G., Neuwinger, J., Bahrs S., Nieschlag, E. (1992). Internal quality control of semen analysis. *Fertil. Steril.*, **58**: 172–178.

Diamond JM (1986). Ethnic differences. Variation in human testis size. *Nature,* **320**(6062): 488–489.

Donovan D.F., DiBaise M., Sparks A.E.T., Kessler J., Sandlow J.I. (1998). Comparison of microscopic epididymal sperm aspiration and intracytoplasmic sperm injection/in-vitro fertilization with repeat microscopic reconstruction following vasectomy: is second attempt at reversal worth the effort. *Hum. Reprod.*, **13**: 387–393.

Dunphy B.C., Kay R., Barratt C.L., Cooke I.D. (1989). Quality control during the conventional analysis of semen, an essential exercise. *J. Androl.*, **10**: 378–385.

el-Borai N., Inoue M., Lefevre C., Naumova E.N., Sato B., Yamamura M. (1997). Detection of herpes simplex DNA in semen and menstrual blood of individuals attending an infertility clinic. *J. Obstet. Gynaecol. Res.*, **23**: 17–24.

Fari A., Vergès J., Trévoux R., Belaisch J. (1976). Examens biochimiques et bactériologiques du plasma séminal humain. I. Méthodologie. Application. Interprétation. *Revue Franç. Gynec.*, **71**(11): 663–674.

Farrer J.H., Walker A.H., Rajfer J. (1985). Management of postpubertal cryptorchid testis: a statistical review. *J. Urol.*, **134**: 1071.

Felder H., Meyer F., Osborn W., Pantke E., Rottgers H., Schultze-Leva A., Brahler E. (1996). Psychological aspects in the therapy of the andrological sterility factor with regard to the unfulfilled wish for a child. *Andrologia*, 1, **28** (Suppl. 1): 53–56.

Ford W.C., Mathur R.S., Hull M.G. (1997). Intrauterine insemination: is it an effective treatment for male factor infertility? *Baillière's Clin. Obstet. Gynaecol.*, **11**: 691–710.

Forman R., Gilmour-White S., Forman N. (1996). *Drug-induced Infertility and Sexual Dysfunction.* Cambridge University Press, pp. 168.

Fraga C.G., Motchnik P.A., Shigenaga M.K., Helbock H.J., Jacob R.A., Ames B.N. (1991). Ascorbic acid protects against endogenous oxidative DNA damage in human sperm. *Proc. Natl. Acad. Sci. USA*, **88**: 11003–11006.

Fraga C.G., Motchnik P.A., Wyrobek A.J., Rempel D.M., Ames B.N. (1996). Smoking and low antioxidant levels increase oxidative damage to sperm DNA. *Mutat. Res.*, **351**: 199–203.

Futterweit W., Mechanick J.I. (1987). Myotonic dystrophy presenting as male infertility: a case report. *Int. J. Fertil.*, **32**: 142–144.

Gerris J. (1997). A comparative investigation into the real efficacy of conventional therapies versus advanced reproductive technology in male reproductive disorders. PhD thesis.

Gerris J., Van Nueten J., Van Camp C., Gentens P., Van de Vijver I., Van Camp K. (1988). Clinical aspects in the surgical treatment of varicocele in subfertile men. II. The role of the epididymal factor. *Eur. J. Obstet. Gynecol. Reprod. Biol.*, **27**: 43–51.

Geva E., Bartoov B., Zabludovsky N., Lessing J.B., Lerner Geva L., Amit A. (1996). The effect of antioxidant treatment on human spermatozoa and fertilization rate in an in vitro fertilization program. *Fertil. Steril.*, **66**: 430–434.

Gilbert B.R., Witkin S.S., Goldstein M. (1989). Correlation of sperm-bound immunoglobulins with impaired semen analysis in infertile men with varicoceles. *Fertil. Steril.*, **52**: 469–473.

Giwercman A., von der Maase H., Skakkebaek N.E. (1993). Epidemiological and clinical aspects of carcinoma in situ of the testis. *Eur. Urol.*, **23**: 104–110.

Glezerman M., Bernstein D., Zakut C., Misgav N., Insler V. (1982). Polyzoospermia: a definite pathologic entity. *Fertil. Steril.*, **38**: 605–608.

Golomb J., Vardinon N., Homonnai Z.T., Braf Z., Yust I. (1986). Demonstration of antispermatozoal antibodies in varicocele-related infertility with an enzyme-linked immunosorbent assay (ELISA). *Fertil. Steril.*, **45**: 397–402.

Guérin J.F., Ben Ali H., Roller J., Souchier C., Czyba, J.C. (1986). Alpha-glucosidase as a specific epididymal enzyme marker: its validity for the etiologic diagnosis of azoospermia. *J. Andol.*, **7**: 156–162.

Hagerman R.J., Amiri K., Cronister A. (1991). Fragile X checklist. *Am. J. Med. Genet.*, **38**: 283–287.

Hargreave T.B. (1994). History and examination. In *Male Infertility*, 2nd ed, ed. T.B. Hargreave. Springer Verlag, London, pp. 17–36.

Hargreave T.B. (1996). Varicocele: overview and commentary on the results of the World Health Organization varicocele trial. *Current Advances in Andrology*, ed. GMH Waits, J Frick, GWH Baker, Bologna Monduzzi Editore, pp. 31–44.

Hausmanowa-Petrusewicz I., Borkowska J., Janczewski Z. (1983). X-linked adult form of spinal muscular atrophy. *J. Neurol.*, **229**: 175–188.

Henkel R., Muller C., Miska W., Schill W.B., Kleinstein J., Gips H. (1995). Acrosin activity of human spermatozoa by means of a simple gelatino-lytic technique: a method useful for IVF. *J. Androl.*, **16**: 272–277.

Homonnai Z.T., Paz G.F., Weiss J.N., David M.P. (1980). Relation between semen quality and fate of pregnancy: retrospective study on 534 pregnancies. *Int. J. Androl.*, **3**: 574–584.

Horvath P.M., Bohrer M., Shelden R.M., Kemmann E. (1989). The relationship of sperm parameters to cycle fecundity in superovulated women undergoing intrauterine insemination. *Fertil. Steril.*, **52**: 288–294.

Imperato-MacGinley J.L., Guerrero L., Gautier T. et al. (1974). Steroid 5α-reductase deficiency in man: an inherited form of male pseudohermaphroditism. *Science*, **186**: 1213–1215.

Jow W.W., Steckel J., Schlegel P.N., Magid M.S., Goldstein M. (1993). Motile sperm in human testis biopsy specimens. *J. Androl.*, **14**: 194–198.

Juul S. (1997) The European infertility and subfecundity study group. Geographical variation of subfertility problems in Europe. *Abstract book of the International Symposium on Environment, Lifestyle and Fertility*, December 7–10 1997, Aarhus, Denmark, pp. 63–66.

Keck C., Gerber-Schafer C., Wilhelm C., Vogelgesang D., Breckwoldt M. (1997). Intrauterine insemination for treatment of male infertility. *Int. J. Androl.*, **20** Suppl 3: 55–64.

Kent-First M.G., Kol S., Muallem A., Ofir R., Manor D., Blazer S., First N., Itskovitz-Eldor J. (1996). The incidence and possible relevance of Y-linked microdeletions in babies born after intracytoplasmic sperm injection and their infertile fathers. *Mol. Hum. Reprod.*, **2**: 943–950.

Kessopoulou E., Powers H.J., Sharma K.K., Pearson M.J., Russell J.M., Cooke I.D., Barratt C.L. (1995). A double-blind randomized placebo cross-over controlled trial using the antioxidant vitamin E to treat reactive oxygen species associated male infertility. *Fertil. Steril.*, **64**: 825–831.

Kholkute S.D., Meherji P., Puri C.P. (1992). Capacitation and the acrosome reaction in sperm from men with various semen profiles monitored by a chlortetracycline fluorescence assay. *Int. J. Androl.*, **15**: 43–53.

Klaiber E.L., Broverman D.M., Pokoly T.B., Albert A.J., Howard P.J. Jr., Sherer J.F. Jr. (1987). Interrelationships of cigarette smoking, testicular varicoceles, and seminal fluid indexes. *Fertil. Steril.*, **47**: 481–6.

Kohn F.M., Schill W.B. (1994). The alpha-sympathomimetic midodrin as a tool for diagnosis and treatment of sperm transport disturbances. *Andrologia*, **26**: 283–387.

Kotoulas IG, Cardamakis E, Michopoulos J, Mitropoulos D, Dounis A (1994). Tamoxifen treatment in male infertility. I. Effect on spermatozoa. *Fertil. Steril.*, **61**: 911–914.

Krause W., Holland-Moritz H., Schramm P. (1992). Treatment of idiopathic oligozoospermia with tamoxifen-a randomized controlled study. *Int. J. Androl.*, **15**: 14.

Kurinczuk J., Bower C. (1997). Birth defects in infants conceived by intracytoplasmic sperm injection. *Br. Med. J.*, **315**(7118). 1260–1265; discussion 1265–1266.

Lahteenmaki A. (1993). In-vitro fertilization in the presence of antisperm antibodies detected by the mixed antiglobulin reaction (MAR) and the tray agglutination test (TAT). *Hum. Reprod.*, **8**: 84–88.

Lai Y.M., Lee J.F., Huang H.Y., Soong Y.K., Yang F.P., Pao C.C. (1997). The effect of human papilloma virus infection on sperm cell motility. *Fertil. Steril.*, **67**: 1152–1155.

Land J.A., Courtar D.A., Evers J.L.H. (1997). Patient dropout in an assisted reproductive technology program: implications for pregnancy rates. *Fertil. Steril.*, **67**: 278–281.

Lissens W., Sermon K. (1997). Preimplantation genetic diagnosis: current status and new developments. *Hum. Reprod.*, **12**: 1756–1761.

Maers E.M. Jr., Stamey T.A. (1968). Bacteriological localization patterns in bacterial prostatitis and urethritis. *Invest. Urol.*, **5**: 492–318.

Mahmoud A.M., Comhaire F.H., Depuydt C.E. (1998a). The clinical and biological significance of serum inhibins in subfertile men. *Reprod. Toxicol.*, **12**: 591–599.

Mahmoud A.M., Geslevich J., Kint J., Depuydt C., Huysse L., Zalata A., Comhaire F. (1998b). Seminal plasma alpha-glucosidase activity and male infertility. *Hum. Reprod.*, **13**: 591–595.

Mahmoud A.M, Schoonjans F., Zalata A.A., Comhaire F.H. (1998c). The effect of male smoking on semen quality, reducing capacity, reactive oxygen species, and spontaneous and assisted conception rates, presentation at Andrology in the Nineties, International symposium on male infertility and assisted reproduction, Genk, Belgium, April 22–25, 1998.

Mahmoud A.M., Tuyttens C.L., Comhaire F.H. (1996). Clinical and biological aspects of male immune infertility: a case-controlled study of 86 cases. *Andrologia*, **28**: 191–196.

Malandrini A., Villanova M., Piomboni P., Collodel G., Spadaro M., Giunti P., Salvadori C., Morocutti C., Guazzi G.C. (1993). Ultrastructural sperm abnormalities and cerebellar atrophy: does a correlation exist? Report of two cases without endocrine hypogonadism. *J. Submicrosc. Cytol. Pathol.*, **25**: 371–375.

Martin-Boyce A., David G., Schwartz D. (1977). Genitourinary infection, smoking and alcohol in the male. *Rev. Epidemiol. Sante. Publique.*, **25**: 209–216.

McClure R.D., Khoo D., Jarvi K., Hricak H. (1991). Subclinical varicocele: the effectiveness of varicocelectomy. *J. Urol.*, **145**: 789–791.

Marsman J.W., Brand R., Schats R., Bernardus R.E. (1995). Clinical and subclinical varicocele: a useful distinction? *Eur. J. Obstet. Gynecol. Reprod. Biol.*, **60**: 165–169.

Meistrich M.L. (1993). Potential genetic risks of using semen collected during chemotherapy. *Hum. Reprod.*, **8**: 8–10.

Mercier S., Bresson J.L. (1997). Analysis of chromosomal equipment in spermatozoa of a 46,XY/47,XY/ + 8 male by means of multicolour fluorescent in situ hybridization: confirmation of a mosaicism and evaluation of risk for offspring. *Hum Genet.*, **99**: 42–46.

Merino G., Carranza-Lira S. (1995). Semen characteristics, endocrine profiles, and testicular biopsies of infertile men of different ages. *Arch. Androl.*, **35**: 219–224.

Micic S. (1987). Incidence of aetiological factors in testicular obstructive azoospermia. *Int. J. Androl.*, **10**: 681–684.

Mieusset R., Bujan L. (1995). Testicular heating and its possible contributions to male infertility: a review. *Int. J. Androl.*, **18**: 169–184.

Moosani N., Pattinson H.A., Carter M.D., Cox D.M., Rademaker A.W., Martin R.H. (1995). Chromosomal analysis of sperm from men with idiopathic infertility using sperm karyotyping and fluorescence in situ hybridization. *Fertil. Steril.*, **64**: 811–817.

Mortimer D. (1999). Structured management for male factor infertility. In *The Male Gamete: From Basic Knowledge to Clinical Applications*, ed. C. Gagnon, Cache River Press, Vienna, IL.

Mortimer, D. (1994). *Practical Laboratory Andrology*. New York: Oxford University Press, 393 pp.

Neuwinger, J., Behre, H.M., Nieschlag, E. (1990). External quality control in the andrology laboratory: an experimental multicenter trial. *Fertil. Steril.*, **54**: 308–314.

Nieschlag E., Behre H.M., Schlingheider A., Nashan D., Pohl J., Fischedick A.R. (1993). Surgical ligation vs. angiographic embolization of the vena spermatica: a prospective randomized study for the treatment of varicocele-related infertility. *Andrologia*, **25**: 233–237.

Nieschlag E., Hertle L., Fischedick A., Behre H.M. (1995). Treatment of varicocele: counselling as effective as occlusion of the vena spermatica. *Hum. Reprod.*, **10**: 347–353.

Nilsson S., Edvinson A., Nilsson B. (1979). Improvement of semen and pregnancy rate after ligation and division of the internal spermatic vein: fact or fiction?. *Br. J. Urol.*, **51**: 591.

O'Donovan P.A., Vandekerckhove P., Lilford R.J., Hughes E. (1993). Treatment of male infertility: is it effective? Review and meta-analyses of published randomized controlled trials. *Hum. Reprod.*, **8**: 1209–1222.

Ombelet W., Bosmans E., Janssen M., Cox A., Vlasselaer J., Gyselaers W., Vandeput H., Gielen J., Pollet H., Maes M., Steeno O., Kruger T. (1997b). Semen parameters in a fertile versus subfertile population: a need for change in the interpretation of semen testing. *Hum. Reprod.*: **12**: 987–993.

Ombelet W., Vandeput H., Janssen M., Cox A., Vossen C., Pollet H., Steeno O., Bosmans E. (1997c). Treatment of male infertility due to sperm surface antibodies: IUI or IVF? *Hum. Reprod.*, **12**: 1165–1170.

Ombelet W., Wouters E., Boels L., Cox A., Janssen M., Spiessens C., Vereecken A., Bosmans E., Steeno O. (1997a). Sperm morphology assessment: diagnostic potential and comparative analysis of strict or WHO criteria in a fertile and a subfertile population. *Int. J. Androl.*, **20**: 367–372.

Padron O.F., Brackett N.L., Sharma R.K., Lynne C.M., Thomas A.J. Jr., Agarwal A. (1997). Seminal reactive oxygen species and sperm motility and morphology in men with spinal cord injury. *Fertil. Steril.*, **67**: 1115–1120.

Pagidas K., Hemmings R., Falcone T., Miron P. (1994). The effect of antisperm autoantibodies in male or female partners undergoing in vitro fertilization–embryo transfer. *Fertil. Steril.*, **62**: 363–369.

Pakrashi A., Chatterjee S. (1995). Effect of tobacco consumption on the function of male accessory sex glands. *Int. J. Androl.*, **18**: 232–236.

Pavlovich C.P., Schlegel P.N. (1997). Fertility options after vasectomy: a cost-effectiveness analysis. *Fertil. Steril.*, **67**: 133–141.

Pierik F.H., Vreeburg J.T., Stijnen T., De Jong F.H., Weber R.F. (1998). Serum inhibin B as a marker of spermatogenesis. *J. Clin. Endocrinol. Metab.*, 83: 3110–3114.

Robertson S, Harrison RF (1984). Secondary Sterility. In *Fertility and Sterility, the Proceedings of the XI World Congress on Fertility and Sterility*, ed. R.F. Harrison, J. Bonnar & W. Thompson Workshop No. 46, p. 461–464, Lancaster: MTP Press Ltd.

Schill W.B., Feifel M. (1984). Low acrosin activity in polyzoospermia. *Andrologia*, **16**: 589–591.

Schill W.B., Topfer-Petersen E., Heissler E. (1988). The sperm acrosome: functional and clinical aspects. *Hum.Reprod.*, **3**: 139–145.

Schlegel P.N. (1997). Is assisted reproduction the optimal treatment for varicocele-associated male infertility? A cost-effectiveness analysis. *Urology*, **49**: 83–90.

Schoysman R., Daniore V. (1991). Artificial insemination for oligospermia. A critical review. *Acta Eur. Fertil.*, **22**: 75–86.

Sexton W.J., Jarow J.P. (1997). Effect of diabetes mellitus upon male reproductive function. *Urology*, **49**: 508–513.

Sharpe J., Skakkebaek N.E. (1993). Are estrogens involved in falling sperm counts and disorders of the male reproductive tract?. *Lancet*, **341**: 1392–1395.

Sigman M., Jarow J.P. (1998). Endocrine evaluation of infertile men. *Urology*, **50**: 659–664.

Skakkebaek N.E. (1978). Carcinoma in situ of the testis: frequency and relationship to invasive germ cell tumours in infertile men. *Histopathology*, **2**: 157–170.

Takihara H., Sakatoku J., Fujii M., Nasu T., Cosentino J.M., Cockett A.T.K. (1983). Significance of testicular size measurement in andrology. I. A new orchiometer and its clinical application. *Fertil. Steril.*, **39**: 836–840.

Tanner J.M. (1962) In *Growth at Adolescence*, 2nd edn, Oxford: Blackwell Scientific Publications.

Testart J., Lassalle B., Frydman R., Belaisch J.C. (1983). A study of factors affecting the success of human fertilization in vitro. II. Influence of semen quality and oocyte maturity on fertilization and cleavage. *Biol.Reprod.*, **28**: 425–431.

Thonneau P., Ducot B., Spira A. (1983). Risk factors in men and women consulting for infertility. *Int. J. Fertil. Menopausal Stud.*, **38**: 37–43.

Thonneau P., Mieusset R. (1997). Occupational heat exposure and male fertility. *Abstract Book of the International Symposium on Environment, Lifestyle and Fertility*, December 7–10 1997, Aarhus, Denmark, p.9.

Topfer-Petersen E., Volcker C., Heissler E., Schill W.B. (1987). Absence of acrosome reaction in polyzoospermia. *Andrologia*, 19 Spec No: 225–228.

Török L. (1985). Treatment of oligozoospermia with tamoxifen (open and controlled studies). *Andrologia*, **17**: 497.

Tournaye H., Lissens W., Liebaers et al. (1997a). Heritability of sterility: clinical applications. In *Genetics of Human Male Infertility*, ed. C. Barratt, C. De Jonge, D. Mortimer, J. Parinaud. EDK, Paris, pp.123–144.

Tournaye H., Staessen C., Camus M., Verheyen G., Devroey P., Van Steirteghem A. (1997b). No evidence for a decreased fertilizing potential after in-vitro fertilization using spermatozoa from polyzoospermic men. *Hum. Reprod.*, **12**: 2183–2185.

Tournaye H., Verheyen G., Nagy P., Ubaldi F., Goossens A., Silber S., Van Steirteghem A.C., Devroey P. (1997c). Are there any predictive factors for successful testicular sperm recovery in azoospermic patients? *Hum. Reprod.*, **12**: 80–86.

Trum J.W., Gubler F.M., Laan R., van der Veen F. (1996). The value of palpation, varicoscreen contact thermography and colour Doppler ultrasound in the diagnosis of varicocele. *Hum. Reprod.*, **11**: 1232–1235.

Tuerlings J.H., Mol B., Kremer J.A., Looman M., Meuleman E.J., te Meerman G.J., Buys C.H., Merkus H.M., Scheffer H. (1998). Mutation frequency of cystic fibrosis transmembrane regulator is not increased in oligozoospermic male candidates for intracytoplasmic sperm injection. *Fertil. Steril.*, **69**: 899–903.

Urry R.L., Middleton R.G., McGavin S. (1986). A simple and effective technique for increasing pregnancy rates in couples with retrograde ejaculation. *Fertil. Steril.*, **46**: 1124–1127.

van der Ven K., Messer L., van der Ven H., Jeyendran R.S., Ober C. (1996). Cystic fibrosis mutation screening in healthy men with reduced sperm quality. *Hum. Reprod.*, **11**: 513–517.

van der Ven K., Peschka B., Montag M., Lange R., Schwanitz G., Van der Ven H. (1998). Increased frequency of congenital chromosomal aberrations in female partners of couples undergoing intracytoplasmic sperm injection. *Hum. Reprod.*, **13**: 48–54.

Vazquez-Levin M.H., Notrica J.A., Polak de Fried E. (1997). Male immunologic infertility: sperm performance on in vitro fertilization. *Fertil. Steril.*, **68**: 675–681.

Vezina D., Mauffette F., Roberts K.D., Bleau G. (1996). Selenium-vitamin E supplementation in infertile men. Effects on semen parameters and micronutrient levels and distribution. *Biol. Trace Elem. Res.*, **53**: 65–83.

Von Eckardstein S., Simoni M., Bergmann M., Weinbauer G.F., Gassner P., Schepers A.G., Nieschlag E. (1999). Serum inhibin B in combination with serum follicle-stimulating hormone (FSH) is a more sensitive marker than serum FSH alone for impaired spermatogenesis in men, but cannot predict the presence of sperm in testicular samples. *J. Clin. Endocrinol. Metab.*, **84**: 2496–2501.

West A.B., Butler M.R., Fitzpatrick J., O'Brien A. (1985). Testicular tumours in subfertile men: report of 4 cases with implications for management of patients presenting with infertility. *J. Urol.*, **133**: 107–109.

Williamson RCN (1976). Torsion of the testis and allied conditions. *Br. J. Surg.*, **63**: 465–476.

World Health Organization (1987). Towards more objectivity in diagnosis and management of male infertility. *Int. J. Androl.*, Suppl. 7.

World Health Organization (1992a). The influence of varicocele on parameters of fertility in a large group of men presenting to infertility clinics. *Fertil. Steril.*, **57**: 1289–93.

World Health Organization (1992b). A double-blind trial of Clomiphene Citrate for the treatment of idiopathic male infertility. *Int. J. Androl.*, **15**: 299–307.

World Health Organization (1993). *WHO Manual for the Standardized Investigation and Diagnosis of the Infertile Couple.* CUP.

World Health Organization (1999). *WHO Laboratory Manual for the Examination of Human Semen and Sperm–Cervical Mucus Interaction*, CUP, 4th edn.

World Health Organization Task Force on Methods for the Regulation of Male Fertility (1996). Contraceptive efficacy of testosterone-induced azoospermia and oligozoospermia in normal men. *Fertil. Steril*, **65**: 821–829.

World Health Organization (1984). Workshop on the standardized investigation of the infertile couple, Moderator P.J. Rowe, Co-ordinator M. Darling. *Proceedings of the 11th World Congress on Fertility and Sterility*, ed. R.F. Harrison, J. Bonnar, W. Thompson, pp. 424–442. Lancaster: MTP Press.

Yavetz H., Yogev L., Hauser R., Lessing J.B., Paz G., Homonnai Z.T. (1994). Retrograde ejaculation. *Hum. Reprod.*, **9**: 381–386.

Yoshida A., Miura K., Shiari M. (1996). Chromosome abnormalities and male infertility. *Assisted Reprod. Rev.*, **6**: 93–99. Quoted from Tournaye et al. (1997a).

Zalata A., Hafez T., Mahmoud A., Comhaire F. (1995). Relationship between resazurin reduction test, reactive oxygen species generation, and gamma-glutamyltransferase. *Hum. Reprod.*, **10**: 1136–1140.

Zalata A., Christophe A., Horobin D., Dhooge W., Comhaire F. (1998). Effect of essential fatty acids and antioxidants dietary supplementation on the oxidative DNA damage of human spermatozoa. *Hum. Reprod.*, 13 (abstract book 1), **R-004**: 270–271. (Abstract).

Index

Printed in the United States
By Bookmasters